Straighter, Stronger, Leaner, Longer

Straighter, Stronger, Leaner, Longer

A Head-to-Toe Strengthening, Stretching, and Pain-Relieving Program

Renée Daniels with Janice Billingsley

AVERY

a member of Penguin Group (USA) Inc.

New York

Published by the Penguin Group
Penguin Group (USA) Inc., 375 Hudson Street, New York, New York 10014, USA ·
Penguin Group (Canada), 10 Alcorn Avenue, Toronto, Ontario M4V 3B2, Canada (a division
of Pearson Penguin Canada Inc.) · Penguin Books Ltd, 80 Strand, London WC2R 0RL,
England · Penguin Ireland, 25 St Stephen's Green, Dublin 2, Ireland (a division of
Penguin Books Ltd) · Penguin Group (Australia), 250 Camberwell Road, Camberwell, Victoria 3124,
Australia (a division of Pearson Australia Group Pty Ltd) · Penguin Books India Pvt Ltd,
11 Community Centre, Panchsheel Park, New Delhi–110 017, India · Penguin Group (NZ),
Cnr Airborne and Rosedale Roads, Albany, Auckland 1310, New Zealand (a division of Pearson
New Zealand Ltd) · Penguin Books (South Africa) (Pty) Ltd, 24 Sturdee Avenue,
Rosebank, Johannesburg 2196, South Africa

Penguin Books Ltd, Registered Offices:
80 Strand, London WC2R 0RL, England

Neither the publisher nor the authors are engaged in rendering professional advice or services to the individual
reader. The ideas, procedures, and suggestions contained in this book are not intended as a substitute for con-
sulting with your physician. All matters regarding your health require medical supervision. Neither the authors
nor the publisher shall be liable or responsible for any loss or damage allegedly arising from any information or
suggestion in this book. The opinions expressed in this book represent the personal views of the authors and not
of the publisher.

Most Avery books are available at special quantity discounts for bulk purchase for sales promotions, premiums,
fund-raising, and educational needs. Special books or book excerpts also can be created to fit specific needs. For
details, write Penguin Group (USA) Inc. Special Markets, 375 Hudson Street, New York, NY 10014.

Library of Congress Cataloging-in-Publication Data

Daniels, Renée.
Straighter, stronger, leaner, longer: a head-to-toe strengthening, stretching,
and pain-relieving program / Renée Daniels with Janice Billingsley.
p.   cm.
Includes index.
ISBN 1-58333-227-8
1. Stretching exercises.   I. Billingsley, Janice.   II. Title.
RA781.63.D36   2005   2004062335
613.7'1—dc22

Printed in the United States of America
1   3   5   7   9   10   8   6   4   2

Photos by Benjamin Oliver
Illustrations by Jan MacDougall
Book design by Mauna Eichner and Lee Fukui

This book is dedicated to all of my clients, students, and patients who taught me that the best and most beneficial path to fitness is an exercise program that is specific to each individual. Their many questions and their search for answers about how to make their own bodies work better are what motivated me to write this book. I realized that if they were so eager for information about healthy exercise, there must be many more people who would benefit from what I teach.

I also dedicate this book to my loving husband, Jason Daniels, who believes in me and has the grace to tell me so.

Acknowledgments

I would like to thank my Equinox family, whose guidance and support helped lead me to this very fulfilling career of medical exercise: my "father in fitness," Bob Esquerre, who started me on the path to fitness training; Rich Baretta, one of the best teachers and trainers in New York City; and Michael K. Jones, RPT, who opened up the world of medical exercise for me. These men taught me that intelligent exercise should be available to everyone.

I am also grateful to Jim Wharton, known as "The Mechanic" for his skill in working with professional athletes, who taught me so much about the science of stretching.

Finally, I would not be where I am today without the influence and teaching of Evie Vlahakis, a New York City physical therapist who took the time to show me how to take care of the body after injury. She taught me patience and persistence and introduced me to the joy of helping people regain their strength and confidence as they recover from injury.

Contents

Foreword

When I went to my local Equinox gym several years ago, I asked to be matched to a trainer who could help me improve my fitness as well as be mindful of a knee injury from which I'd recently recovered. I expected, as had been my experience, to find a competent fitness professional who would walk me through a series of standard exercises that would strengthen and tone my muscles. I would trust my own medical training to protect me from hurting my knee again.

Instead, I met Renée.

From the moment she introduced herself and we began to talk, I realized that she was different from any other trainer I'd ever had. I was amazed by how knowledgeable she was about anatomy and body function, comparable to any physical therapist. When I asked her about it, she told me she had a certification in medical exercise and had spent seven years as a physical therapist's assistant, unheard of in a fitness trainer.

She thoroughly understood the problems with my knee, and it was extremely satisfying to me as a physician to be able to communicate on such a professional level and so easily with someone about my health concerns and fitness goals.

As we began working together and Renée put me through some exercises, she asked me how I spent my day, how much time I spent at a desk (a fair amount), what sports I played (tennis), and other questions that I now understand are key to her program of creating a functional exercise program tailored to an individual's lifestyle.

She explained that I had slightly rounded shoulders, most probably from working at my computer, and needed to do some exercises to improve my posture. She also said that I would benefit from some core exercises that would strengthen my stomach, back, and hip girdle and ease pressure on my knee joints. Finally, she recommended a series of knee exercises to strengthen all the muscles surrounding my knee equally so I would lower my risk for further knee injury.

This was light-years away from my experience with any of the other half dozen trainers I'd had over the years, who concentrated on how much better I could look with toned biceps and tight abs but never talked about exercising my body for how I used it.

When we began training together, I continued to be impressed by all Renée brought to her work. She had been a dancer, so understood movement and the importance of flexibility, alignment, balance, and proper technique during exercise. She had used those skills in conjunction with her experience in physical therapy and fitness training to develop an enormous repertoire of exercises to build strength and endurance and increase flexibility of all the muscle groups.

I found it extraordinary how she was able to tap into this extensive knowledge base to design an exercise program that suited my particular needs. Clearly, she has an unusual talent for three-dimensional visualization and instant recall.

After several months of training with Renée, my posture improved, I became much stronger, and I found that I had stopped worrying about my knees. I felt better, found my daily tasks, from carrying a suitcase to reaching for something on the top shelf, easier to perform, slept better, and must have looked better, because friends kept telling me so.

I looked forward to our sessions because I always learned something new about how my body worked. Whenever I asked why we were doing an exercise, Renée would explain exactly what muscles I was working (by name) and why it was important to do so. I don't know if I was the only one who did this—perhaps I'm more inquisitive because of my medical background—but I found it fascinating to relearn biomechanics in a nonacademic setting.

Which brings me to another quality I appreciate in Renée—her attentiveness. From our first meeting throughout the time we trained together, Renée listened very carefully to what I told her about my workouts, answered all my questions, and was diligent in monitoring me during our training sessions. Before each session began, she would ask me questions—"How do you feel?" "Do any muscles hurt?" "Any lasting pain?"—to evaluate the effectiveness of my previous workout. Furthermore, she was able to modify or adjust an exercise to build on my progress from session to session or to take into account a temporary setback or muscle strain.

She is a stickler for proper technique, explaining that poor form not only renders an exercise inefficient but can cause injury. Often we would repeat an exercise several times until I understood how to do it properly and why it was important.

I'm now very aware of the importance of my posture and do simple shoulder exercises several times a day when I've spent a long time at my desk. I understand the importance of conditioning my body for whatever activities I do, especially when tennis season rolls around.

And I, too, have become a stickler for proper exercise technique. It's all I can do at the gym sometimes not to tap a fellow athlete on the arm to tell him that he's doing his chest presses incorrectly.

When Renée told me she was writing a book about her exercise program that would contain all the terrific exercises she knows, I was both elated and skeptical. Elated because I would have in hand all the wonderful information she shared with me, but skeptical because how could she possibly convey her enthusiasm, personal warmth, and expertise to readers who couldn't experience her program in person?

I need not have worried. In straightforward, easily understandable prose that echoes Renée's manner with her clients, *Straighter, Stronger, Leaner, Longer* helps the reader to analyze how she uses her body every day and to design a personalized program to improve how she moves. This is a terrific book for anyone who wants basic, easily presented information about how her body works and how to make it work better.

TERRY FONVILLE, M.D.
Department of Medicine, St. Vincent's Hospital
and Medical Center, New York City

Introduction

When I was in my twenties, I was a professional dancer in New York City and assumed I was in great shape. I was slim, supple, and graceful, and worked very hard at my craft. Anyone looking at me would have thought I was in excellent physical condition.

But one day I was doing a basic dance step, which involved standing on one leg and arching my back as far as I could, when I felt a sharp pain in my lower back. I was sore but not worried. I just went home a little early to rest for the next day.

That day's rest turned into almost four months of agony as I learned I had a slipped disc in my lower back and began a long journey back to health and to a new way of thinking about body fitness.

What I learned during my rehabilitation was that as a dancer, I had been trained for flexibility, balance, and range of motion, but had been taught absolutely nothing about muscle function or the importance of training the muscles of the core to prepare my body for my rigorous work. I realized that it was most likely the weakness of those muscles that had led to my back injury.

The more I learned about strength training and the importance of functional exercise, the more I wanted to know, so I stopped dancing and began a new career in fitness training.

I was lucky to join Equinox gyms at the inception of the Equinox Fitness Training Institute. Studying with well-known experts in the fitness field like Bob Esquerre and Rich Baretta, I immersed myself in anatomy and biomechanics with an emphasis on medical exercise so I could train people with injuries like the one I had suffered.

I was able to observe operations at a local hospital so I understood how, for instance, a knee replacement surgery was done, and saw firsthand the trauma of surgery, which made me sensitive to the needs of people who came to the gym following surgery.

After being certified as a trainer and receiving an additional certification in medical exercise through the American Academy of Health, Fitness and Rehabilitation Professionals, founded by my teacher, Michael K. Jones, RPT, I began to apply what I'd learned in my classes and with my personal clients. Along with their fitness training, I taught them about their anatomy so that they understood why I recommended the exercises I did, and why it was important to develop a personalized program to strengthen and increase the flexibility of their muscles for their own daily activities.

During this time, I began to volunteer at the physical therapy clinic that was part of the gym. I wanted to learn more about rehabilitation from the physical therapists, which I certainly did over the seven years I was there. But I was also able to teach something to the therapists, because I knew so many exercises from my dance and fitness work. As a result, they began to ask me to help them create specialized exercise programs for their patients with some of the many exercises I used with my regular clients.

Eventually I became the fitness training manager at my Equinox gym so that I could teach other trainers about the benefits of teaching their clients how to take charge of their bodies in the same way.

I feel very fortunate that my training in the three disciplines of dance, fitness training, and physical therapy has given me an unusual set of skills to benefit my clients. I help them analyze their own movement by teaching them about their anatomy, I explain body mechanics to them so that they understand how their bodies actually move, and I teach them exercises to enhance these movements safely and efficiently.

If they are recovering from an injury, I can help them understand why they might have become injured in the first place and help them create an individualized exercise program to prevent a recurrence of their pain and improve their strength, flexibility, and function.

But perhaps most important, what I teach them gives them the confidence to take charge of their own fitness in a way they've never done before. They learn how to pay attention to how they move, and to make sure they exercise to keep themselves strong and flexible for whatever activities they do.

It is this system that I can offer to you.

This book is arranged simply to help you get the information you need as easily as possible. The first two chapters give an overview of your anatomy, an explanation of how my system has helped some of my clients, and information on how to do a self-assessment of your own body's strengths and weaknesses.

Subsequent chapters each cover a different part of the body, discussing the most common problems I see among clients, explaining simple anatomy, and giving you exercises that will increase the strength and flexibility of your muscles so that you will function better.

Next is a chapter that gives you two menus of exercises to use as the basis of your own program.

You can read the whole book, you can jump to the chapter that deals with your back pain, or you can skip to the exercises.

It gives me great pleasure to watch clients slowly shed their bad habits and begin to appreciate how efficiently and beautifully their bodies function while they improve their posture and balance, strengthen their muscles, and become more flexible. They smile more and exude a new confidence. Their friends ask them if they've gotten a haircut or lost weight, telling them there's "just something different" about them. And, of course, there is. They're in charge of their bodies, and it shows.

I hope the same will happen to you.

Straighter, Stronger, Leaner, Longer

1

What Your Body's All About

Forget BMWs and Porsches. If you want to see a really beautifully designed machine, look in the mirror. There isn't anything like the human body for efficient movement combined with stability. You've got an ingenious skeletal system that provides structure and a musculature system that provides the strength for you to move it around. The body is both simple and complex, like any exceptionally creative work of art.

And yet what I hear most from a new client is that his or her body *doesn't* work. A young, active man will tell me that when he lifts weights, his shoulder hurts. A middle-aged, healthy woman is upset that she can work in her garden for only a short time before her back begins to ache. An older man can't figure out why his knees bother him after simply walking down the stairs at home.

They know something's wrong, they are very frustrated that they have no answers, and they want to feel good again so they can remain active.

Some clients assume their discomfort is caused by stress, others by the fact that they're getting older. Some are convinced that a recent event, such as moving their sofa when the rug was being cleaned, is the reason they're in pain.

I explain that these conditions can of course contribute to discomfort or pain. Accidents and congenital problems, which are out of anyone's control, can also certainly be the reason for injury.

But for the majority of my clients, the underlying reason for their physical problems is this: Their daily activities and bad postural habits, repeated every day for weeks, months, and years, have created alignment problems and muscle weaknesses that have slowly undermined their alignment and made them ripe for the pain they suffer.

Because they don't know that their poor body habits, from the way they sit at work to the way they hold their babies, are the most likely reason for their discomfort, they do little or nothing to exercise the body to be strong enough for how they move every day. This is the primary reason why they suffer from so many aches and pains.

When I explain this to my clients, it's as if I'm telling them for the first time that the earth is round. They have no idea that there is any connection between poor postural habits and their discomfort. The idea that a shoulder problem is more likely related to poor posture from years of bending over the computer all day than to the tennis game they played over the weekend astounds them.

But this is a very logical concept. It makes sense that when you perform the same tasks every day, sometimes for years, they will have an impact on your body. If you have been sitting at your desk at work with your upper body rotated toward your computer, your muscles have tightened and affected the alignment of your trunk. This unnatural posture has created imbalances in the strength and flexibility of your muscles—some are too tight, others have become weak. As a result your joint movement has been compromised and your muscles have become strained, which can lead to pain.

While to anyone with a background in anatomy this ignorance of basic mechanics seems surprising, I think there are two important reasons most people are unaware of the connection between the way they use their bodies every day and the aches and pains they may be suffering.

First, our bodies usually get us where we want to go and allow us to get through the workday and perform well enough for most of our recreational activities. As a result, we take our ability to move for granted and don't pay much attention to our bodies until they start to hurt.

Second, even if you are interested in improving your fitness, there's very little information available to laypeople about simple body mechanics and why it's important to maintain strength and flexibility for what they do. As a result, many people are left with outdated fitness information that doesn't address their needs.

But I have found that if I can teach my clients the basics of anatomy so that they understand body mechanics, teach them to analyze how they use their own bodies during the day, and then teach them exercises that address their individual needs, they become strong and flexible so that all their activities become easier. They no longer have pain at work or at play.

Further, as they become more knowledgeable about body mechanics and how they use their own bodies, they begin to understand what exercises they need to do to keep healthy for their activities.

They begin to take charge of their own fitness and health in a truly remarkable way.

When you understand how your body works, you will have the tools to create a personalized exercise program that will keep you strong, flexible, and less prone to injury.

My program isn't a cure-all for everyone, and I don't want to offer facile advice to people suffering from serious pain due to illness or trauma. But for people who are able to participate in regular exercise, my program works. Intelligent exercise need not be the province of a few expert exercise gurus. We all deserve a shot at it.

BODY MECHANICS 101

Everyone knows a little bit about body mechanics, or at least thinks he does. We know we should have good posture—head up, shoulders back, spine straight. Add to that an increasing number of people, often those who take Pilates, who know the importance of strengthening the muscles of the core. And there are many people who enjoy yoga and have learned how to stretch their muscles to increase their flexibility and movement.

However, most people are often quite unaware of the most basic facts about their anatomy—their skeletal system, the importance of their joints, how their muscles work.

Nor do they understand how the body actually moves. And finally, no one has ever explained to them the connection between how they use their bodies every day and its effect on their posture.

But you don't need a degree in kinesiology to understand your anatomy, body mechanics, and the importance of good alignment and strong and flexible muscles and how to achieve them. I teach these things to my clients every day. The practical information I give them becomes part of a personalized exercise plan that helps them strengthen their muscles and improve their posture, with the result that they reduce or eliminate their pain and feel better than they have in a long time.

So let's begin at the beginning.

THE SIX SEGMENTS OF THE BODY

Think of the little square wooden blocks you played with when you were small, and imagine stacking them in a neat tower. That's how your body is arranged, in separate segments: the head, shoulders, trunk, pelvis, knees, and ankles.

When Segments Are in Alignment

When all the segments are stacked neatly one on top of the other, like the blocks, you have a perfectly aligned body. Each segment works alone and in conjunction with the other segments, enabling your joints to move without stress or pain. You can move your trunk and all your extremities efficiently in all directions. It's a beautiful thing.

And very rare.

Very few people have perfect alignment. Some athletes, dancers, and people aware of the importance of posture and alignment come close. They have the fluid synchronicity that comes with good alignment, and they are easy to spot because they move so easily and gracefully. You're not sure why, but they just look good.

When Segments Are out of Alignment

Unfortunately, many of us are a collection of precariously stacked blocks about to topple over if the wind changes. Rounded shoulders, swaybacks, hyperextended knees, and forward-tilting heads are all signs that the segments of your body aren't lined up properly, and that your alignment is not what it should be.

When your segments are out of alignment there's sort of a trickle-down effect throughout your whole body during movement. Every time you move, the other key components of your body, such as your muscles, joints, ligaments, and tendons, all try to compensate for the imbalances caused by the misalignment of the primary postural groups. This is outside of their job description, however, so while they give it their best shot, they can't keep you from injury. Muscles become overstretched or tightened; ligaments and tendons become strained; bursae sacs get compressed while trying in vain to stabilize your joints so that you can move the way you'd like. It's basically a mess in there.

There's no need to despair, however, because exercise can help you redress the imbalances you've created. But first you should know how your segments stack up.

THE PLUMB LINE

You can figure out for yourself if your segments are lined up properly and if you are unnecessarily making yourself vulnerable to injury, not to mention looking older than you have to. To do this you can do the same thing doctors and physical therapists do when assessing their patients: check your posture against the plumb line.

What Is the Plumb Line?

The plumb line is used by health professionals to determine whether you have good body alignment. Proper alignment means that you have good posture, which allows you to move

Figure 1.1

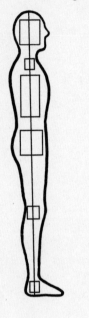

with maximum efficiency and minimal stress on the muscles and joints. The plumb line measures your posture against a postural grid of this optimal stance.

Stand sideways in front of a full-length mirror, or ask a friend to look at you sideways, to see how your posture measures up against the ideal plumb line.

This is what you're looking for: Your ear, shoulder, hip, knee, and ankle joints should be stacked, one on top of the other, with the plumb line running through the center of the joints (see Figure 1.1). If this is how you look it means your regular postural stance is close to your natural plumb line. This is terrific because your alignment and posture are as good as it gets, anatomically speaking. Being in line with gravity is key to efficient body mechanics, because gravity is a strong force acting on your body, and you want to work with it rather than against it. The less you mess with its potent force, the easier it is to move the way you want to.

Figure 1.2

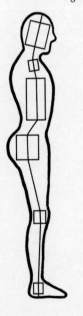

How Do You Assess Your Plumb Line?

If your plumb line looks a little wavy, don't despair. Most people's posture doesn't follow the plumb line. Your ears might be several inches in front of your shoulders, your shoulders in front of your hips, or your knees extended back behind your hips (see Figure 1.2).

All these positions, which are very common, could indicate that something has gone wrong with your posture and you are making movement harder than it has to be by putting unnecessary stress on your joints and the muscles, as well as the ligaments and tendons that surround them. The upshot is that you're setting yourself up for discomfort, lack of mobility, and eventual injury.

Tracing your plumb line and discovering any imbalances gives you your own personalized postural grid, so you can assess your posture and detect any misalignments that can cause potential injuries. Then you can figure out what areas you need to work on.

Now that you have a basic understanding of the segments of your body and why it's important for them to be in alignment, it's time to learn a little bit about the muscles, which are the heroes of good posture. As you read further and understand what your muscles are up to, you'll be able to do exercises tailored to your own situation so that your posture will improve and you will look and feel better.

MAGIC MUSCLES

I have great respect for muscles, and when you understand how they work and what they do for you day after day without complaint, you will, too.

How Muscles Hold You Up

First and foremost, your muscles hold you up. There are hundreds and hundreds of them throughout your body, and they support your skeleton. Without your muscles, you would simply crumple to the floor. I'm always surprised at how many of my clients don't know this simple, crucial fact about their bodies. I don't know if people have seen too many Halloween skeletons, which seem to jerk around on their own, and assume that's how their own bones work, or, more likely, they've simply never thought about it, but it's important to know that your muscles are what get your bones moving.

How Muscles Act as Anchors

Second, muscles protect and stabilize your joints. Shoulders, hips, elbows, knees, and ankles are all insulated by layers of smooth, supple muscles that surround your joints and provide a safe cushion for them. They are more than just a cozy covering, though. The muscles that surround your joints, when strong, hold the joints in place so they can do their jobs of allowing you freedom of movement, and at the same time protect them from injury. If you exercise and strengthen these muscles, it is like having an insurance policy for your joints, keeping them safe and healthy as you get older.

How Muscles Allow You to Move

Third, muscles allow you to move. Every move you make is possible because sets of muscles, called *opposing* muscle groups, work in tandem to create movement. In order for your hand to bring a glass of water to your mouth, your biceps are contracting at the same time that your triceps are stretching. Walking up the stairs? You are contracting the quadriceps muscles on the top of your thighs and simultaneously stretching the opposing set of muscles, your hamstrings, which are at the back of your thighs. This alternate stretching and contracting of muscle groups in synchrony governs all your movements and gives you an exceptional range of motion. Without this ingenious system, you'd be lurching around like Frankenstein.

Now it's time to move from what your muscles do for you to what you can do for your muscles.

NORMAL RESTING LENGTH

The way to better alignment and posture is to return your hardworking muscles to their *normal resting length* between movements. This phrase sounds deceptively easy, like all you have to do is get out the popcorn, sit on the sofa, watch television, and rest your muscles. Sorry.

What Normal Resting Length Means

The normal resting length of a muscle is the length of the muscle when no force is being applied to it, when it's quietly resting after, say, you've played a mean tennis match. It means that muscles return to their proper length after movement. They are not stretched out; they aren't too tight. Like toned athletes, they are primed and supple, healthy and ready for their next assignment.

In a perfect world, all muscles would be in their normal resting length right now and you wouldn't have to worry about it. In fact, if your posture is good and your body properly aligned, your muscles will have no problem returning to their normal resting length after any movement.

When Your Muscles Aren't in Their Normal Resting Length

But most of us aren't so lucky. Many things conspire against normal resting length. Poor posture and repetitive work habits are two of the more common causes. Tension can cause some muscles to become permanently shortened. The effects of injury and surgery compromise muscle length. Even just sitting at a desk all day creates weaknesses in muscles because they simply don't get the use they should.

If you don't exercise your muscles properly to compensate for all the above, they eventually become so stressed that it's very hard for them to return to their normal resting length over time. This happens very often in the workplace. If you spend most of your day bent over a computer, the muscles along your upper back are continually stretched out and become elongated and weak. Similarly, if you cradle a phone to your ear all day, the muscles on one side of your neck are contracting all the time and become tight and lack flexibility.

When normal resting length is compromised, efficient joint motion is sacrificed. In addition, the muscle imbalances begin to put too much stress on the ligaments and tendons that surround the muscles, which leads to injury and pain.

You can see and feel the results of these muscle imbalances. You develop rounded shoulders. Your neck muscles are so tight that you can't rotate your head. Your posture suffers and your alignment is poor. You look older than you should.

So, to feel and look better, begin to think how you use your body and how that affects your posture. Second, analyze how your daily activities affect your movement, and what other factors, such as tension, injury, or pain, could be contributing to muscle imbalances, which in turn have affected your alignment.

To do that, the next chapter will help you to analyze how you use your body in your daily activities and how your habits could be creating muscle imbalances. You will then be able to identify what parts of your body might need special attention in order to improve your posture and alignment.

2

How Your Everyday Movements Affect Your Body

have a good friend who's an actress and who's in great shape, but a few years ago she began complaining to me that her left ankle was very sore and caused her pain when she walked. This is someone who works out regularly and is very aware of her body—she's an actress, after all—but she couldn't figure out what was wrong and neither could I.

Then I finally went to see her in a long-running play she'd been appearing in. I watched her in one scene where she sat for about fifteen minutes with her legs crossed, right foot and ankle wrapped around her left foot and ankle like a pretzel. Bingo!

It turned out she sat that way every day for her scene, and the extreme torque she'd created in her foot and ankle had caused the muscles around her ankle joint to become terribly overstretched, compromising their ability to stabilize the ankle joint and resulting in the pain she felt. When I told her the probable source of her trouble, she stopped crossing her ankles during the scene, did some exercises I gave her to strengthen her ankle, and she was fine.

It's hard to believe that doing something for fifteen minutes a day can throw you out of whack, but it happens all the time. Activities and habits that seem harmless enough in themselves can, when repeated over time, slowly erode the normal resting length of your muscles and, eventually, compromise your alignment. Most people aren't aware of this, and even if they recognize that something's wrong, they lack the knowledge to figure out what the problem is and what to do about it. But if you take the time to think about how you use your body every day, you can take the first step toward body awareness so that you can improve your strength, flexibility, and range of motion.

This is what I do with my clients and what you can learn to do for yourself.

DAILY ROUTINES

My first meeting with clients includes a physical assessment so I can design a safe and personalized program for them. But also important is to ask clients how they use their bodies on a daily basis. I want to know how they're sitting, standing, turning, bending, lifting, and reaching throughout the day. All these movements indicate what muscles clients are using, or not using, and gives me the information I need to help them address any aches and pains they may be having. No matter what you do every day, from teaching nursery school to playing the cello, you are using some muscles more than others, and you need to understand how that affects your body and could be causing you problems.

So my questions include: What's your job? Is it active or sedentary? Are you sitting at a desk all day, or standing at work, or driving in a car? In that job, how do you spend most of your time—at a computer, standing at a counter, carrying your baby around the house? On a scale of one to ten, how stressful is your work? (Everyone knows this!)

The answers give me the information to design an exercise program that takes into account what muscle groups need strengthening, others that need stretching, and where to work on improving a client's range of motion. But equally important, answering the questions makes people, often for the first time, really think about how they use their bodies and begin to understand how their daily activities are affecting them and are perhaps even the source of their discomfort and sometimes fatigue.

CLIENT STORIES

Before you try to analyze how your own activities may be causing you trouble, it might help to know the stories of some my clients—why they came to me and how they got back in shape by using my program.

Reading about them will help you think about your own daily activities and how your movements affect how you look and feel.

LESLIE

Leslie is a successful clothing designer in her mid-forties who was a Pilates refugee. She had signed up for Pilates classes to improve her strength and flexibility, but found that doing some of the exercises hurt her neck and shoulders, so she was referred to me because of my medical exercise background. She wanted relief from her pain, particularly in the neck, and to lose weight and regain her energy level.

To look at her, you'd be surprised that Leslie was having all these problems. Though somewhat overweight, she looked generally healthy. Further, although it was stressful, she enjoyed her job and worked hard at it. But it was precisely the requirements of her job that were the primary source of her trouble.

When people think of physically demanding jobs, they think of moving men hauling sofas down a flight of stairs or construction workers scrambling around a job site, but Leslie's job, as are many office jobs, was as hard on her body as the most strenuous outdoor work.

First of all, she spent a good part of the day on her feet, standing at her drawing board, and the effects of gravity on her body were a primary source of her discomfort. People don't often think of the earth's gravitational pull as affecting their bodies, but in exchange for keeping us from flying into space, gravity can put a lot of stress on your body, and standing upright for long periods of time takes energy and strength. In Leslie's case, being on her feet all day and the extra weight she was carrying around were major causes for her fatigue.

Second, although she walked around in her office at work, most of the time she was standing bent over a drawing board as she drew sketches, her trunk leaning forward and her head tipped down over her work.

Leslie had no idea that her daily habits were the cause of her physical troubles, however, and didn't know that increasing the strength and flexibility of the muscles she used at work would significantly reduce her pain. Instead, she turned to Pilates to feel better.

The problem she faced, however, was that many of the postures Leslie was asked to do at her Pilates class were difficult or impossible to execute due to her already weak and stressed upper body. The Pilates workout, for instance, includes a lot of rolling up through the spine, starting with the head and neck, and since Leslie's neck and shoulder muscles were so weak, she didn't have the strength to do this movement without terrible neck pain.

Also a factor for Leslie was that when she was under stress, she took it in her shoulders, which worsened the pain in her upper body. Everyone responds to stress physically, whether they know it or not. Many people, like Leslie, unwittingly pull their shoulders up around their ears when tense. Others take tension in their backs, or internally, in their stomachs. No matter how you manifest stress, it has a deleterious effect on your body.

Leslie needed an individualized exercise program that focused first on strengthening her weakened shoulder and back muscles and stretching the tight muscles of her chest and neck, then on improving her posture and alignment and strengthening the muscles of her core. I also prescribed an aerobic program to help her lose weight. Finally, I taught her some exercises she could do at work during the day to alleviate the physical impact of her job.

After training for several weeks, the first thing Leslie noticed was that she no longer had neck pain, which motivated her to continue her workouts. As she continued her program, her posture and upper body strength improved dramatically, and she lost weight, felt more energetic, and was pain-free.

In addition to working out at the gym, she began to do back- and neck-care exercises at work to relieve the tension caused by leaning over her drawing table.

Now Leslie understands the importance of paying attention to how she moves throughout the day and knows what exercises she can do to manage any discomfort at work. She can continually adjust her exercise program based on her daily activities so that she maintains her alignment, posture, and strength and flexibility.

DAVID

David was one of my more reluctant clients. In fact, the only reason he came to me was because his doctor insisted he learn some exercises to strengthen his back muscles to help alleviate chronic back pain.

But as far as David was concerned, even though his back bothered him quite a bit throughout the day, his heat therapy and regular cortisone shots kept him well enough to play his thrice-weekly golf games, a sport to which he was passionately devoted.

In his assessment, I learned that David, in his early fifties, was a successful businessman who traveled a lot in his job and, though quite slim, did no regular exercise. Most of his work-day was spent sitting down, at a desk when he was in his office, on a plane during trips and at meetings and conferences he attended out of town.

This explained his back problems in a nutshell. David spent most of his day sitting, which strained the muscles in his lower back. He admitted that whenever he stood up from a chair, his muscles were stiff and painful.

This sedentary lifestyle causes problems on its own, but David was exacerbating his back troubles with his frequent golf games. A golf swing uses the whole body, from the legs through the hips, then through the trunk of the body, the upper body, and finally the arms. The torque needed to hit a clean, hard ball demands a lot of power and stability in the hips, trunk, and shoulders. If these muscles aren't strong, they will become strained by the repetitive motion of a golf swing and, for some, cause serious injury.

But David, like many recreational golfers I work with, didn't really think of golf as a sport that needed physical preparation. To him golf was primarily a mental game, almost like chess. He was absorbed by the challenge of getting the ball to the right place on the fairway and dropping in putts on the green. He explained to me, in fact, how he prepared mentally for his matches by clearing his mind so he could focus on his shots. But, perhaps because golf is a leisurely sport and he didn't perspire, he didn't think he needed any physical preparation. All he did, he told me, was twist his body from side to side a few times while waiting to tee off on the first hole.

I explained to him the damage he was doing to his back, by both his lack of exercise and playing golf without conditioning his body. He lacked strength and muscular endurance, and when muscles get tired, they get tight, causing pain. Strengthening and restoring flexibility to muscles of his trunk would not only free him from pain but probably improve his golf swing. But to do so, he would have to stop playing golf for a few weeks while he began to strengthen and restore flexibility to his muscles.

David was appalled. It was one thing to begin an exercise program to alleviate his pain, and anything that could improve his golf game was good, but he hadn't bargained on having to actually abstain from his favorite pastime. It was as if I'd told him he had cancer.

But eventually, and unhappily, he agreed that spending the rest of his life depending on cortisone shots and heat therapy for relief from back pain was probably not the smartest idea, so we began training together twice a week.

At first a large part of his workout consisted of deep stretching exercises, as his back and shoulder muscles were extremely tight, and soon we began a program to gradually strengthen the muscles that had caused him such discomfort. Once the flexibility in his back had improved, and he was no longer in pain, we began to concentrate on his overall conditioning to improve his posture and alignment and increase his strength so he would be less likely to face injury as he got older.

But I emphasized to David that his training always had to

support his activities. As long as his job was sedentary and he continued to play golf, he needed to pay special attention to exercises that strengthened his lower back and abdominal muscles.

I also taught him some simple stretches to do throughout the day to relieve the tension in his back that he felt at work. This is a great way to keep strong and prevent problems from occurring. It also helps remind people to pay attention to how they use their bodies at work and play.

David, once my most resistant client, has become one of my most ardent fans, which I like to think is because of the success of the program I designed for him rather than the fact that his handicap has dropped by several points since he started working with me.

EVE

Eve came to me for the reason a lot of my clients do—she wanted to get in shape and look buff. In her thirties, with two young children at home, she had recently finished physical therapy for a shoulder injury and wanted to get back to training. Before her shoulder injury, she had swum for exercise, but had to stop because she could no longer raise her right arm above her head without discomfort. Now her shoulder felt better, and she wanted to resume exercising.

She liked swimming, but didn't want to hurt her shoulder again. Also, she didn't understand how she had hurt it in the first place, so she asked me if I could design a fitness program for her to follow up her physical therapy and help her avoid future injury.

When we talked and I tested Eve's fitness level, I saw that she was a healthy and active woman. Chasing after two small children gave her plenty of exercise. Unlike David and Leslie, the least of her worries was being sedentary during the day. Her eating habits weren't the best, as she tended to snatch food on the fly, another common trait of busy mothers, but her weight was okay. However, she was not particularly strong, and I saw that her posture was poor and her right shoulder was slightly higher than the left.

I explained that it was these last three factors that, combined with her swimming, had probably caused her shoulder injury.

Recreational swimming is great exercise to build cardio-vascular strength and muscular endurance, but it isn't a complete exercise and does nothing to improve posture and alignment. If a swimmer isn't strong and well conditioned throughout her whole body before she swims, the repetitive movements in the swim stroke will gradually strain her muscles, creating overuse injuries.

This is what had happened to Eve. Delighted to be on her own and doing something for herself, yet on a tight schedule, she regularly jumped right into the pool and began her laps with no warm-up or strength training. Her right side was stronger than her left (everyone is dominant on one side of the body) so she unwittingly worked that side the hardest. In addition, the mechanics of her stroke were poor.

Eve was fascinated to have this explained to her, especially when I told her that if she committed herself to a well-rounded strength program, combined with flexibility and range-of-motion exercises, she not only could resume swimming with ease but would look sensational.

Because my main focus is on body mechanics and making sure a client exercises with good form, I tend not to dwell on the aesthetic rewards of my program. But people who follow my program are always reporting back to me that people notice how much better they look.

Eve was a good example. I designed a program for her that first focused on correcting her shoulder alignment, which included exercises to strengthen her core. After about two months, she had lost some weight and her posture had improved dramatically as she had gained strength in her upper body. She had also gotten quite buff.

She was happy that she could return to swimming again, but was equally delighted with how she looked. She told me gleefully one day that a friend of her daughter's had referred to her as "the pretty mommy."

MAXWELL

Another one of my younger clients who was getting himself into trouble with his exercise was Maxwell, a self-described "gym rat," whose regular workouts at the gym made him look strong and fit.

In his twenties, Maxwell was a salesman who spent up to five hours a day behind the wheel of his car. He thought that working out at the gym was making up for all the time he spent driving, but he didn't know that his daily activities were putting specific stresses on his body and that the exercises he was doing were exacerbating those stresses rather than relieving them.

Although he was quite strong, Maxwell was very stiff—he had trouble getting out of bed in the morning—and the exercises he did at the gym were hurting his shoulders rather than making them feel better.

After he told me about his job and showed me his workout routine, I explained to him that driving for long periods of time with his arms elevated at the steering wheel put a lot of stress on his neck and shoulders. Also, sitting in a car in the same position for long periods of time is very hard on the body—it simply gets tired of holding the same position and tightens up, which was what was causing the stiffness in his back.

In addition, Maxwell was performing some of his exercises incorrectly at the gym. When he did bench presses, he lowered his arms too far. When he worked at the lat pull-down machine, he lowered the bar behind his head rather than to the top of his chest. Both of these exercises strained different muscles in his shoulders and caused him pain.

So while Maxwell was diligent in wanting to take care of his body, he was doing himself more harm than good.

Once he understood that the way to pain-free fitness was to incorporate into his program exercises that managed the tension in his back, and to learn the proper exercise techniques, he was eager to get started on my program.

First, I taught him stretches to relieve the pain in his back and neck, and then we worked on a program of exercises to improve his shoulder alignment and posture so that his workouts included ways to compensate for the rigors of his car-bound job.

Next I helped him design a program for the road, so that he could stop during the day, get out of the car, and do some simple stretches to alleviate the strain he was putting on his body.

Maxwell still looks like that well-built, buff man who came to me a year ago, but now he feels as good as he looks.

ALLEGRA

One of my most challenging clients was Allegra, a violinist who performs internationally, has recorded numerous CDs, and teaches the violin in New York City.

She was referred to me by her physical therapist after she had dislocated her shoulder during a yoga class. It is bizarre to think that someone could incur a serious injury in a yoga class, because yoga is a terrific conditioning program that relieves tension and tones the body.

But Allegra shouldn't have been in the class in the first place because, although she didn't know it, she was suffering from a repetitive stress injury in her shoulder caused by her constant stroking of the violin bow. Her shoulder muscles were already very stressed, so when she tried to hold a dynamic yoga pose with her shoulder, the effort was too much for her weak muscles and she dislocated her shoulder.

She was panicked because she had an important concert booked in France six months down the road and had to be rehearsed and ready to go in time. Her physical therapist was helpful in working on her shoulder, but she needed an exercise program that would keep the shoulder strong and prevent another injury.

In her assessment, I saw that she played the violin with her shoulders elevated around her ears, so that when she stroked her bow, she was using the muscles around her neck rather than the lower shoulder muscles that anchor the shoulder. In addition, she did no strengthening exercises for the muscles that surrounded her shoulder joint. The combination of her tight neck muscles and the weak muscles in her shoulder had contributed to a serious misalignment of her shoulder joint. Because of this, she was ripe for injury, so that even a yoga exercise was enough to cause a shoulder dislocation.

When I explained this to her, she immediately wanted to learn exercises to strengthen her weak muscles and improve her shoulder alignment and range of motion so she could stroke her bow without pain. I designed a strength and flexibility program for her that she followed religiously.

She was strong and healthy by the time her concert date approached, and was so impressed with the program I gave her that she has sent a number of her fellow violinists to me to help them prevent the kind of injury she suffered.

HOW DO YOU USE YOUR BODY?

Recognize yourself in any of my clients? Look through the questions below for more help in thinking about how you use your body and any potential problems you might be creating in the way you spend your days. I've grouped the questions by the corresponding parts of your body so you can go to the chapter dealing with that area to learn more about any problems you have.

Head and Neck

1. Is your head tilted forward?

2. Do you have loss of range of motion in your neck in any direction?

3. Do you have any neck pain?

4. Do you spend more than a half hour at a time on the phone without using a headset?

5. Do you spend a lot of time looking down to read or type at your keyboard?

Shoulder

1. Do you have pain between your shoulder blades?

2. Do your shoulders roll forward?

3. When you stand in a relaxed position, are the palms of your hands facing back?

4. Is the bottom of your shoulder poking out?

5. Can you lift your arm over your head and to the side without pain?

6. Do you tend to carry stress in your shoulders?

7. Is your computer set up in an ergonomically correct position?

8. Do you carry a heavy purse or satchel over one shoulder?

Back

1. Do you sit at your desk with your upper body rotated toward your computer screen?

2. Do you spend a lot of time driving a car?

3. Do you have any lower back pain?

4. Do you lean forward when you walk, like a coach?

Hips

1. Do you stand on your feet all day at work?

2. Do you have a rolling gait, like a cowboy?

3. Is it hard for you to sit cross-legged on the floor?

4. Look at the heels of your shoes. Are they worn down on one side or the other?

Knees

1. Does it hurt to walk up or down stairs?

2. Have you had knee surgery?

3. Do you avoid exercises that strain your knees, such as squats?

Ankles

1. Do you have pain when you step on your heel?

2. Do you fall over on your ankles?

3. Do you have trouble balancing?

Arms and Wrists

1. Do you have a radiating pain that travels down your arm?

2. Do you have pain when you bend and straighten your arms?

3. Have you ever had tennis elbow?

4. Do you work at the computer without a wrist pad?

5. Do you have trouble opening a jar?

3

The Core—
Control Central
for Your Body

Thanks to growing interest in Pilates and yoga, most people have heard of the core. Pilates, particularly, focuses on exercises to strengthen the muscles of the core, muscles its founder, Joseph Pilates, calls "the girdle of strength."

But I find that while many of my clients have been told that a strong core is important to fitness, they really don't understand what that means.

They have little idea about the anatomy of the core, why strong core muscles are so crucial to efficient, pain-free movement, and how core muscles work closely with the other muscles of the body to share this work. Further, because no one has taught them the importance of a well-rounded core exercise program, their workouts tend to focus on aesthetics rather than on function, and are not as comprehensive or effective as they could be. The result is that weak core muscles are very common among my clients and one of the main reasons why they often experience discomfort in their daily activities.

THE CORE OF THE CORE

Most people know by now that the core includes more muscles than the rectus abdominus, the muscles you exercise for a flat tummy. They understand that the core refers to the entire musculature surrounding the spine, pelvic girdle, and hip.

But they need to know that the reason we have all these muscles in the core is that they are involved in every movement you make.

What have you been doing today? Driving your car, looking over your shoulder when you changed lanes, reaching into the glove compartment to get your sunglasses? Cooking dinner, bending down to get a pan out of the cupboard, opening the refrigerator to get the milk? Making a presentation at work, standing in front of a room, turning toward the video screen to explain the slides you're showing?

Each of these movements—bending, lifting, reaching, leaning back and forward, rotating your torso—relies on the muscles of your core. This is because the core muscles hold the spine and hip in place while you move, keeping all the other postural groups of the body in alignment, including your shoulder and hip girdles. The ability of the core muscles to stabilize your trunk also allows them to absorb a great deal of the force placed on the body during movement.

When the core muscles are weak, however, they are unable to do either of these jobs, forcing the other muscles in the body to pick up the slack. When this happens, the muscles outside the core, no matter how strong, become fatigued and strained. As they tire, the muscles become tight, which puts undue pressure on your joints, making movement less efficient if not impossible. Tight muscles also cause pain. In fact, much of the pain that my clients feel can be traced to overall weakness of the core muscles.

The good news is that a good core exercise program can dramatically reduce pain and discomfort and as dramatically improve how you look and feel.

Knowing a little bit about the muscles of the core and how crucial they are to efficient movement will help you understand why fitness professionals are always touting the importance of the core and will also motivate you to make core exercises a priority in your fitness program.

Stabilizing Muscles

There are two sets of muscles in the trunk. One set is the deep muscles that are very close to the bones of the spine and hip. These muscles are crucial to stabilizing your spine so that you can move efficiently. They are also rarely exercised. When I explain this to my clients and teach them exercises to strengthen their deep core muscles, they are truly amazed at how much stronger they become. Their daily tasks are easier to accomplish, their balance improves, and they begin to really enjoy how their bodies move.

Figure 3.1

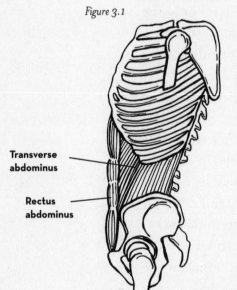

Transverse abdominus

Rectus abdominus

These muscles include: the transverse abdominus, the internal obliques, the lumbar multifidus, and the muscles of the pelvic floor. The transverse abdominus (see Figure 3.1) is particularly important because as it contracts to compress and stabilize the spine, it automatically activates several other core muscles to do the same, helping to maintain good alignment and absorbing the force of the body while other muscles are executing movement.

Superficial Muscles

More familiar to most people is the second set of core muscles, the superficial muscles. These are the muscles that actually create movement. Some are the ones you can see when you look in the mirror, like the external obliques, which allow you to rotate your trunk and move it from side to side, and the rectus abdominus, which enables you to bend over. Others, not visible but equally important, are the iliopsoas muscles, which you use when you flex your hip, and the erector spinae muscles.

In a comprehensive exercise program, you exercise both of these muscle groups to increase your strength and stability.

WEAK CORE MUSCLES

Most of my clients who have weak core muscles have no idea that they do. In fact, they've become so accustomed to moving without the benefits of core strength that they're astonished by how much better they feel and how much more efficiently they perform their daily activities after they begin a core-strengthening program.

One of my clients is a 23-year-old woman who swam in college and looks slim and very fit. She mentioned almost casually that after running on the treadmill she always felt pain in her lower back. She assumed she simply had a "bad back" and seemed resigned to endure her pain as the price of fitness.

I explained to her that her back was fine but that her core muscles were weak. When she ran, her muscles couldn't maintain the stability her body needed for optimal movement, and this resulted in strain on her muscles and joints, which caused her pain.

When she began a program to strengthen her core muscles and stretch her lower back, her back pain disappeared completely.

Equally problematic are clients who mistakenly think they understand the importance of the muscles of the core and that they are exercising these muscles properly.

My client Larry was a young man who was very serious about his workout program. He used the machines at the gym, lifted weights, ran on a treadmill, and did at least 100 crunches about four times a week. If you asked him if he was exercising the muscles of the core he would assure you that he exercised these muscles regularly.

But he didn't. He had never been taught that core exercises included more than crunches, so he was using this outdated information as a basis for his workout. As a result, he did no exercises to strengthen the muscles of the core and wasn't nearly as strong as he thought he was. When I tested his overall strength in his assessment, he was amazed and more than a little frustrated to discover that he couldn't do the simplest exercises I gave him for the core, exercises that measure strength, balance, and the ability to stabilize the trunk during movement.

Further, he had very poor posture, leaning forward when he walked. This was an indication that his body was out of alignment and thus prone to injury. This can also be a sign of a weak core.

STRONG CORE MUSCLES

All my clients become experts in the core muscles, even if they don't want to! By explaining basic anatomy and teaching them exercises that strengthen their core muscles, they can't help but appreciate what their core does for them.

The two things I emphasize in my core training, and in all my programming, are exercises that replicate actual movement and the importance of technique.

Functional Exercise

My fitness program focuses on teaching people to take charge of their bodies by learning about their own body mechanics and creating an exercise program that strengthens their body for whatever they do. I've found this to be the most successful way to help my clients become healthy and remain active. Many of my exercises are done in a standing position and are quite dynamic, engaging several muscle groups simultaneously, because that's how you use your body.

This is especially helpful in training the core muscles, because my clients are often unaccustomed to training for daily movement. With my exercises, they learn that core muscles are used every time they perform an activity and can greatly enhance the efficiency of that movement.

A good example is the upright rotation exercise in this chapter (see page 40), a standing exercise that strengthens the muscles that rotate the trunk along with muscles that stabilize the shoulders.

Technique

As important as the exercises that make up a workout program is the way you do them. Proper technique is very important, not only for the core but for all the muscles of the body. There is a clear right way and many wrong ways to do every exercise, and when you execute an exercise with poor form, you won't derive any benefits from it.

Larry told me in his assessment, for example, that he could do 100 sit-ups at a time with no problem, so when we finished our conversation and went into the gym to begin our training session, I asked him to show me his sit-ups.

It turned out that Larry was using his head, shoulder, and arm muscles rather than his stomach muscles to propel himself off the floor. Further, he was pulling himself nearly upright with each crunch, which is much too high. To isolate the stomach muscles during sit-ups, you only need to lift your upper body to a 45-degree angle off the floor. (See Figure 3.2.) When you go any higher than that, like Larry was, you're using your hip muscles, not your stomach muscles.

Figure 3.2

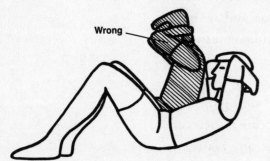

Wrong

When I showed him how to do a sit-up properly so that the exercise concentrated wholly on the right muscle group, he could do only twenty sit-ups. But the good news, I told the embarrassed Larry, was that those twenty sit-ups were strengthening his abs far more effectively than the 100 so-called sit-ups that he had wasted so much time executing.

Larry's regimen also illustrates that less is sometimes more when it comes to exercise. Never sacrifice form for an increase in repetitions of an exercise, because it's then that you get sloppy and negate the benefits of the exercise. Worse, you are putting yourself at risk for injury. Good technique ensures a safe and effective workout.

CORE EXERCISES

Following are the basic core exercises I teach my clients. They work, often in tandem, all the muscles of the core, giving you a sound foundation for all the other exercises you do. Doing them regularly will improve your ability to control your body, your coordination, and your balance.

Not only that, as your core becomes stronger, you will feel more in tune with how your body works. You will automatically begin to use the muscles of your core when you do other exercises and notice quite an improvement in how you function, both at the gym and throughout the day.

You should do core exercises three times a week to build up your strength. You can pick any three to do at each session, but make sure at least one is a standing exercise because these exercises really help your daily functioning.

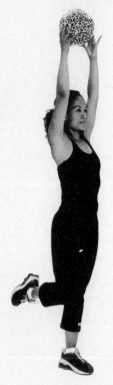

Trunk Flexion

This is a "standing crunch" that strengthens your stomach muscles.

1. Stand upright with legs hip-width apart and arms overhead. With both hands hold a light weight (four pounds is good) or a ball. Lift your right foot so that you're balancing on your left leg. (See Figure 3.3.)

2. Roll forward, bringing hands to the floor, using your stomach muscles rather than the leg and ankle muscles to maintain balance. (See Figure 3.4.) Then round back up.

3. Do three repetitions of 10 on each leg.

IMPORTANT: Concentrate on using your stomach muscles to do the exercise and keeping your shoulders down and relaxed as you bend down. If you have trouble keeping your balance, it's okay to touch the toe of your raised foot to the ground to regain your equilibrium.

Figure 3.3

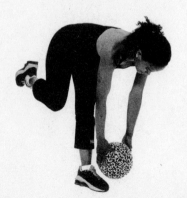

Figure 3.4

Lateral Flexion

This exercises the transverse abdominus.

1. Stand upright, legs hip-width apart.

2. Hold a towel or rope overhead, as shown, with arms shoulder-width apart. (See Figure 3.5.)

3. Lean as far to the right as possible, keeping your stomach pulled in and shoulders relaxed. (See Figure 3.6.)

4. Return to upright position.

5. Do three repetitions of 10.

6. Repeat on the left side.

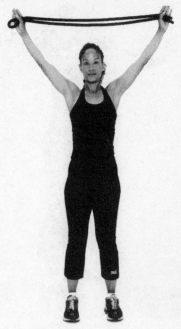

Figure 3.5

IMPORTANT: Think about maintaining good posture while you do this, keeping your butt tucked in and your shoulders back, not rounded forward.

Progression: When you are stronger you can do this exercise on one leg, remembering to keep the ball of your foot flat on the floor—don't put all your weight on your pinkie toe!

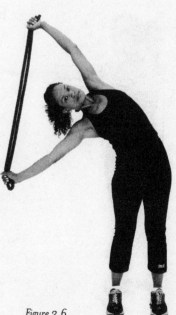

Figure 3.6

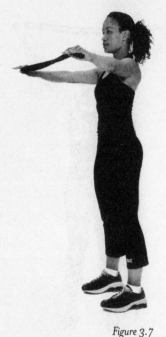

Upright Rotation

This exercises your obliques and other primary core muscles.

1. Stand, legs hip-width apart, arms in front of your body, chest-high and shoulder-width apart, holding a rope or towel. (See Figure 3.7.)

2. Pull stomach in tight and rotate your body to the right as far around as you can, lifting the heel of your left foot as you go and pivoting on the ball of your foot into the movement. Keep your right foot still and stable during the pivot. (See Figure 3.8.)

3. Do three repetitions of 10 on each side.

4. Repeat on the left side.

Figure 3.7

IMPORTANT: Keep your body in a neutral position by making sure your butt isn't sticking out.

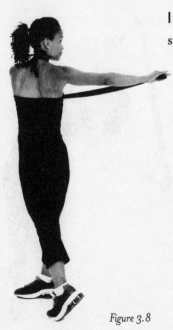

Figure 3.8

Diagonal Trunk Rotation on the Physio Ball

This exercises the whole trunk.

1. Sit on the physio ball so it supports your lower back, arms supporting your head. Lean your body back at a slight angle above the ball. (See Figure 3.9.)

2. Lift your shoulders up and off the ball. Using your stomach muscles, rotate your trunk to the left, reaching your right arm toward your left knee. Your left hand remains supporting your head. (See Figure 3.10.)

3. Do three repetitions of 10 each.

4. Repeat on the left side.

IMPORTANT: Concentrate on using your stomach muscles in this exercise rather than your upper body.

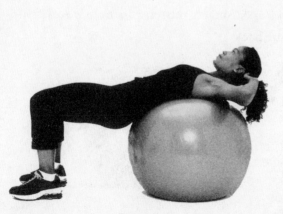

Figure 3.9

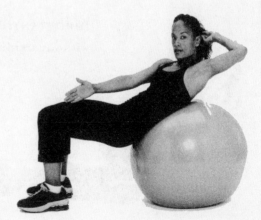

Figure 3.10

Lying Trunk Rotation

This exercise strengthens the obliques and rectus abdominus and other small muscles that stabilize the spine.

1. Lie on your back, with feet on the floor and knees bent.

2. Keeping left knee bent, straighten right leg out and hold below the left knee.

3. Place your left hand out to the side; use your other hand to support your head. (See Figure 3.11.)

4. Flex trunk up and rotate it toward your left knee. (See Figure 3.12.)

5. Lift your trunk up higher, continuing to rotate toward the bended knee, and try to touch your right elbow to the left knee.

6. Do two sets of 10 repetitions each.

7. Repeat on the other side.

IMPORTANT: Use your stomach muscles to help you lift up without arching your back.

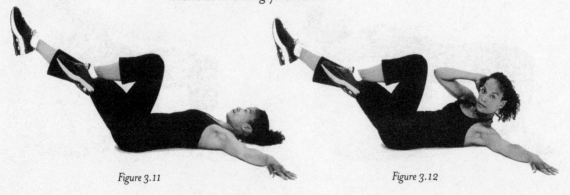

Figure 3.11   *Figure 3.12*

Hook Lying

This exercises the lower abdominal muscles and the muscles of the pelvic floor.

1. Lie on the floor on your back, with your knees bent and feet on the floor. Reach your arms straight out toward the wall behind you.

2. Pull your stomach in as tightly as possible so there is no space between your spine and the floor. This is called a pelvic tilt. (See Figure 3.13.)

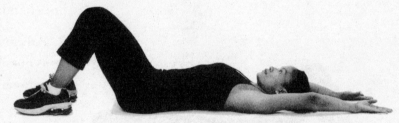

Figure 3.13

3. Keeping your arms straight, lift your head, neck, and shoulders off the floor until your hands touch your knees. (See Figure 3.14.)

4. While maintaining the pelvic tilt, do 10 crunches. Return to the supine position.

5. Do three sets of 10 repetitions each.

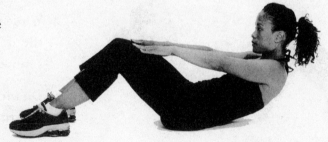

Figure 3.14

IMPORTANT: Keep shoulders and neck relaxed and stomach muscles pulled in so that the spine stays flat on the floor.

Hook Lying Progression

When you feel stronger, you can do this exercise with a five-pound weight or a four-pound medicine ball.

1. Lie on the floor on your back, knees bent, feet on the floor. Reach your arms out straight toward the ceiling, holding the weight or ball with both hands. (See Figure 3.15.)

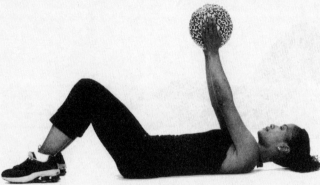

Figure 3.15

2. Pull your stomach in as tightly as possible so there is no space between your spine and the floor. This is called a pelvic tilt.

3. Keeping your arms straight, lift your head, neck, and shoulders off the floor until your hands or ball touch your knees. (See Figure 3.16.)

4. While maintaining the pelvic tilt, do 10 crunches. Return to supine position.

5. Do three sets of 10 repetitions each.

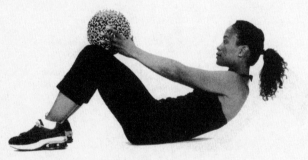

Figure 3.16

Spine Stabilization with Physio Ball

This exercise strengthens the rectus abdominus and the small muscles that stabilize the spine.

1. Kneel in front of the physio ball, arms extended with hands on top of the ball.

2. Slowly lean forward toward the ball, pulling in your stomach muscles as you go. (See Figure 3.17.) Go as far as you can without arching your back.

3. Roll back to upright position.

4. Do three repetitions of 10 exercises each.

IMPORTANT: Keep your body straight and stomach muscles tight.

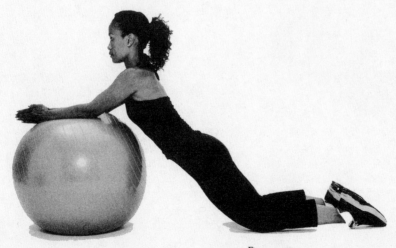

Figure 3.17

4

Get Backs
Back in Shape

Without question, these are the two most common words I hear from my clients: back pain. So many people suffer from this malady that it's a wonder anyone gets up in the morning.

Their experiences mirror national statistics, which state that 80 percent of the American population will experience back pain at some point in their lives and that back pain is second only to the common cold as the reason for days lost at work.

My clients could care less about the statistics. They all come to me with two questions: What is wrong with my back? And how can I fix it?

Many of them have already been to the doctor for back pain. There are many medical reasons for back pain, such as serious injuries to the back, anatomical problems, a disease like scoliosis or herniated and ruptured discs, all of which require a doctor's care.

For those clients, I am often the stop that follows physical therapy. They want to start an exercise program to stay healthy after recovering from surgery or rehabilitation.

But many of the people who come to me have gotten a clean bill of health from their doctors and their backs still hurt. They're frustrated, mystified, and desperate for answers so they can feel better.

What they need more than anything else is information.

THE WAY WE HURT OUR BACKS

Back pain often comes on suddenly, erupting out of nowhere when you're doing nothing more than making your bed or standing up from your desk. You assume that whatever you just did is the reason your back hurts, but that's rarely the case. Most of the back pain I see in my clients isn't because of a specific activity but rather is a result of the way they've been using their bodies over a period of time. Before you blame your household chores for your back pain, see if your habits match those of any of my clients.

Being Active but Deconditioned

A twice-weekly tennis player who also regularly exercised at the gym, Carol was convinced she was in good shape and so was very perplexed as to why she had back pain after her tennis games.

When I asked about her exercise program, I knew why she was having trouble. While she took body sculpting classes that included upper body and leg work, she did no exercises for her core or back muscles, except sit-ups, so these muscles were weak, and her posture and alignment were poor. When she lunged and pivoted on the tennis court, she put tremendous strain on the weakened muscles, and they became very tight, which was what caused her back pain.

Further, her exercise program didn't include a sustained cardiovascular workout, a key component of a comprehensive fitness program. Because of this, her muscles weren't getting a sufficient supply of oxygen and other nutrients when she played tennis, so she had poor stamina and her muscles were stiff. Combined with the fact that she was slightly overweight, which put extra pressure on her joints and ligaments, it was no surprise that Carol suffered from back pain.

It was hard to persuade Carol that her fitness program was not working for her because she'd been doing it for so long and because no one, including her exercise instructor, had ever explained movement and the importance of functional exercise to her.

What finally convinced her to try something new was when I took her downstairs to the rehab center in the basement of our gym and showed her, using a small skeleton we keep on display, the mechanics of movement of the spine and surrounding muscles and why it was important for those muscles to be strong and flexible so she could move without pain. When she could see for herself how stretching and strengthening her trunk muscles would improve how she moved and decrease the incidence of back pain, she was at last willing to start my program.

I have many clients like Carol, who are committed to taking care of their bodies and think they are exercising and staying active for good health, but who are not in good physical condition. Despite their best intentions, their activities unwittingly put them at risk for injury. When they change their programming, they see dramatic results.

Sedentary Lifestyle

Paul was another client with back pain, but for the opposite reason, which was that he had an entirely sedentary lifestyle. He spent almost his whole day in a seated position—in the car driving to work, at work, and at home in the evening watching television.

Since he did no strenuous exercise and wasn't overweight, he was puzzled and frustrated that he was in such pain. He could barely get out of bed in the morning.

But Paul didn't know that probably the biggest source of back pain in our country today is due to simply sitting on our butts. When people think of using muscles, they logically think of movement. And we do use our back muscles all the time when we're moving around—bending, reaching, and lifting. But our back muscles are still working even when we are sitting at a desk all day, driving a car, or tucked in an easy chair in front of the television. Even though we aren't moving, the back still must bear the weight of the entire upper body and stabilize the spine so that we can remain upright. This takes a tremendous amount of strength. In fact, the back muscles actually work harder when we are seated than when we are standing, because when we're on our feet our weight is distributed more evenly throughout the body, lessening the load on the back.

Paul never did exercises to strengthen the muscles of his back and core, and as a result, his trunk was very weak. Sitting put enormous strain on the muscles, which became very tight. This tightness restricted blood flow to the muscles and discs and created terrible back pain.

As I did with Carol, I showed Paul exactly how his spine and the surrounding muscles work and the importance of strengthening the muscles he used most often so that they could handle the jobs he gave them. Once he got over his amazement that simply sitting around all day demanded a great deal of muscle strength and endurance, he, too, began a program to strengthen and stretch the muscles of his back, and his back pain disappeared.

Muscle weakness due to sedentary lifestyles like Paul's has become one of the leading causes of back pain in our country. Yet it could be eliminated quite simply if people did two things: exercise to strengthen their back muscles for the work they do and stretch tight back muscles to return them to their normal resting length. Increasing strength and flexibility boosts endurance, minimizes the compression on the spine, and relieves tension on the muscles. Back pain would be a distant memory.

Muscle Overuse

Forcing muscles to work past their limit of strength and flexibility is another common cause of back pain. Trying to keep up with the person next to you in an exercise class or with the teacher is one way people get hurt. Jumping onto the tennis court or playing a round of golf on the first nice day in spring without doing any conditioning beforehand is also a frequent reason for back pain.

Poor Exercise Programming

Many people are proud of how many abdominal crunches they can do. But doing a lot of sit-ups at the gym without exercising the back muscles creates a serious imbalance of strength of the muscles of the trunk, which support the spine.

A good example of this is an exercise that calls for bending at the waist, reaching for your toes, and then rotating your torso from side to side. To do this exercise without hurting yourself, you need to have a balance of strength between your stomach and back muscles and good flexibility. If you have weak stomach muscles, which many people do, or back pain, you should not do this exercise.

Improper Exercise Technique

Not targeting the right muscles when you work out, or using poor form that strains the muscles rather than strengthening them, is another cause of back pain.

A popular exercise called back hyperextension is a common example of this. It is done on an apparatus at the gym where you tuck your heels on a slight ramp and rest your hips on a pad. Crossing your arms on your chest, you lean forward, stretching the muscles of the back.

To complete the exercise correctly, you pull your upper body back to the point where your shoulders are aligned with your hips. However, many people swing up too far, lifting their body beyond their hips, which can compress the spine and put pressure on the discs.

Picking up heavy objects the wrong way can also cause injury. When you pick up something heavy, hold it as close to your body as possible, bending your hips and knees as you lift. If instead of using your lower body, you keep your legs straight and bend only from the waist, you will put unnecessary pressure on your muscles, joints, ligaments, and discs and could hurt your back.

Poor Circulation

Many of my clients with back pain have given up aerobic exercise altogether because every move they make is agony. They don't understand that inactivity and lack of cardiovascular fitness only increases their pain, restricting the blood flow to the very muscles that need oxygen and other nutrients to function properly. Also, by not moving at all, their muscles have become very tight, causing them even more pain.

GETTING YOUR BACK BACK

The first step in back pain relief is learning to appreciate your muscles. By strengthening them and keeping them flexible, as well as improving your cardiovascular activity, you will get better. Next, it helps to be familiar with all the components of your back. Most likely you've never heard of many of the muscles in your back, what your discs actually do, where your sacroiliac is. But all these parts of your body are toiling away and holding you up as you read this. When you understand how well your body can function when your muscles are strong and flexible, you will be very motivated to start a new exercise program.

WHAT HAVING A BACKBONE REALLY MEANS

The back pain I see in almost all my clients is due to a series of fairly specific muscle imbalances in the trunk: weak abdominal muscles; weak gluteal muscles, which are the muscles of the butt; tight hamstrings; and weak hip flexor muscles.

Many people have heard of these muscles but have no idea how they fit into the grand scheme of back movement. So I always teach my clients the basics about their spine so they can understand exactly how their backs function and why their muscles are weak.

The Spine, Pelvis, and Sacroiliac Joint

It's easy to think of the spine as a straight ramrod that runs down your body from neck to hips, sort of like the pointer your teacher used at school.

But in fact the spine is a wonderfully flexible bony structure that has a gentle "S" curve, allowing you the freedom to move in any way you choose. It is made up of 33 small, bony segments called vertebrae, and is divided into four sections that, starting from the neck down, are called cervical, thoracic, lumbar, and sacrum. In a healthy spine the vertebrae are aligned so that the spine moves easily and efficiently.

At its base in the lower back, the spine lies alongside the pelvis, creating the sacroiliac joint, which enables the spine to move.

In between each vertebra is a disc, an oval, soft piece of cartilage called the annulus fibrosus, filled with a gel-like substance that acts as a cushion between each vertebra, enabling flexible movement of the spine. (See Figure 4.1.)

Figure 4.1

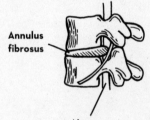

Keeping these discs healthy is extremely important in preventing back pain. Of all the components of the back, the discs are among the most vulnerable to injury. Doctors tell us that discs degenerate as we age, naturally losing some of their elasticity and health, but that isn't the only, or even the primary, reason for disc degeneration.

For the majority of people, no matter how young, disc degeneration begins with poor body conditioning. Weak muscles are unable to do the job of protecting the spine and ligaments, especially when you perform strenuous tasks. This creates a domino effect on your whole body. The weakened muscles become very tight and strained, which in turn restricts blood flow through the muscles to the discs. The discs are then deprived of the nutrients usually carried to them by the blood, nutrients they depend on to maintain health.

It is when this situation continues over time that the discs become vulnerable to the injuries we all know:

Segment instability: Strain on the muscles due to tightness pushes the segments of the spine out of alignment, causing pain during movement. The muscle strain and tightness also limit joint movement, which causes stiffness and poor range of motion.

Herniated disc: The outer covering of the disc, called the annulus fibrosus, becomes weakened and stretched so that the disc bulges in certain spots. The bulges can press against the ligaments and nerves that surround the vertebrae, causing pain. (See Figure 4.2.)

Figure 4.2

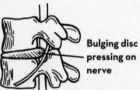

Bulging disc
pressing on
nerve

Ruptured disc: The annulus fibrosus actually tears open so that the gel-like fluid leaks out, pushing through the ligaments to the nerves that also surround the vertebrae, causing radiating pain. This pressure on the nerves is also known as sciatica.

Disc problems are not inevitable, however. Maintaining good muscle tone and flexibility in the back ensures blood circulation to the discs, keeping them healthy and significantly retarding the degeneration process, so that you can function well into old age.

Figure 4.3

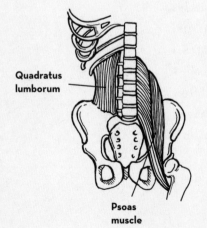

Quadratus
lumborum

Psoas
muscle

Muscles of the Back

The spine is surrounded by many ligaments and muscles that support it and give you the ability to move your back. These muscles, including the quadratus lumborum, erectus spinae, multifidus, and psoas, are deep muscles that are attached to the spine and hip and are crucial to movement and stabilization.

Particularly important to a healthy back are the psoas muscles (see Figure 4.3), two long, thin muscles that run from just under your rib cage down the front of your vertebrae to inside each hip. These muscles help you walk and touch your toes. Two of the most important postural muscles in your body, they help to stabilize the spine and are also responsible for navigating the hip.

When the psoas muscles are weak and tight, which is unfortunately most of the time in many people, trouble begins. In fact, weak psoas muscles combined with weak abdominals are one of the main reasons people have swaybacks, a major cause of lower back pain and segment instability.

Weak and tight muscles are also a contributing factor to trigger point pain that can strike suddenly and be debilitating. When a muscle becomes very tight, blood flow to the muscle is restricted. Without blood, which carries oxygen the muscle needs to remain healthy, the muscle fibers tighten into small nodules that cause pain.

Muscles of the Core

Also important for healthy back muscles is a strong core. In fact, you can't really talk about back muscles without also referring to the core, which is crucial in helping the back muscles stabilize the spine when you move. The combination of strong abdominal and back muscles ensures that you will be able to move easily through your daily activities. A strong trunk also automatically lengthens your spine, which, in addition to making you look thinner and taller, decompresses the vertebrae and eases tension in the back.

CARDIOVASCULAR EXERCISE

Less understood is the key role cardiovascular exercise plays in healthy backs. People think of aerobic exercise as important for weight control and heart health, but its benefits also include pain management. An efficient cardiovascular system allows the blood to move easily through the musculoskeletal system, carrying with it oxygen and other nutrients needed by the body to function. Sustained cardiovascular exercise also helps the muscles become limber and releases endorphins into the body, which are proteins released in the brain through the nervous system. These endorphins have natural pain-relief properties that play an important role in pain management for both episodic and chronic pain.

Every program to reduce back pain must include cardiovascular exercise along with strength and flexibility training.

BACK EXERCISES

If you're suffering from back pain, help is at hand. Even if you don't have back pain, you can benefit from understanding how the back works and why it's important to improve the strength and flexibility of your back muscles. Almost everyone, from weekend basketball players to gym rats to mothers running around after their kids all day, suffers from some muscle imbalances in the trunk area.

The following exercises will provide safe and effective programming for both stretching tight, painful back muscles and strengthening smaller, stabilizing muscles to prevent injury. Done in conjunction with the core exercises in chapter 3, they will significantly relieve troublesome back pain and prevent further pain and injury.

Stretching Exercises

If you are presently suffering from back pain, you should concentrate first on these stretching exercises, which help relax your muscles and guide them back to their normal resting length.

Trunk Flexion Stretch

This is a good stretch for the muscles of the lower spine.

1. Sit on the floor with your knees bent, feet flat on the floor. Grab the top of your shoes with both hands, with your knees just outside your shoulders. (See Figure 4.4.)

2. Keeping your knees upright at 12 o'clock, pull your upper body forward toward your feet, bending your elbows as you pull forward.

3. Tucking your head down so that the top of your head is aimed at the floor, flex your spine forward as far as you can. (See Figure 4.5.)

4. Hold for a count of three. Repeat five times.

IMPORTANT: Keep your knees pointing toward the ceiling to ensure that you stretch your spine.

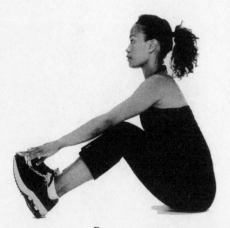

Figure 4.4

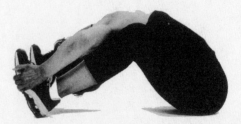

Figure 4.5

Quadratus Stretch on Physio Ball

This exercise stretches the muscles of the back.

1. Sit on the physio ball, pulling your stomach in and holding your chest up. Lift your right arm up. (See Figure 4.6.)

2. Reach over and try to touch your left knee or ankle, leaning your head toward your left knee as well. (See Figure 4.7.)

3. Hold for three seconds. Repeat five times.

4. Repeat exercise, leaning to the other side.

IMPORTANT: Maintaining your balance on the physio ball might be difficult at first, so go only as far as is comfortable while keeping your balance on the ball.

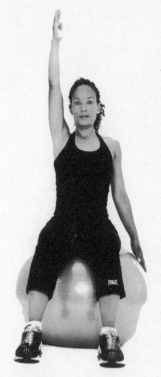

Figure 4.6

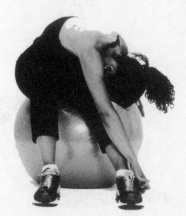

Figure 4.7

Hip Flexor/Psoas Stretch

This is an important exercise to stretch this often tight muscle and return it to its normal resting length.

1. Kneel on one knee beside your bed or a physio ball, resting your arm on the bed or ball and keeping your other foot on the floor. (See Figure 4.8.)

2. Tuck your butt into a pelvic tilt and lean forward on the right leg, feeling the stretch in the front of the left leg thigh. (See Figure 4.9.)

3. Hold for three seconds. Repeat five times.

4. Switch legs and repeat exercise.

IMPORTANT: Maintain your pelvic tilt throughout the exercise so that you are isolating and stretching the psoas muscle.

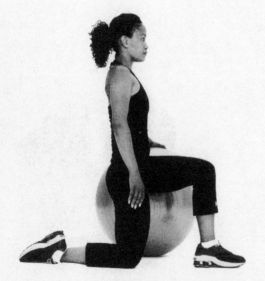

Figure 4.8

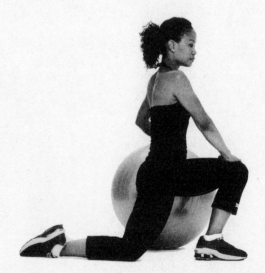

Figure 4.9

Quadratus Stretch

A good stretch for all the back muscles.

1. Sit on the floor, right leg straight in front of you, left leg also on the floor and bent at the knee so that your left foot lies against your right knee. (See Figure 4.10.)

2. Lift your left arm over your head and reach for the outside of your right foot, feeling the stretch along your left side, the site of the quadratus lumborum. (See Figure 4.11.)

3. Hold for three seconds. Repeat five times.

4. Repeat exercise on the other side.

IMPORTANT: Go only as far as is comfortable. Your flexibility will increase over time.

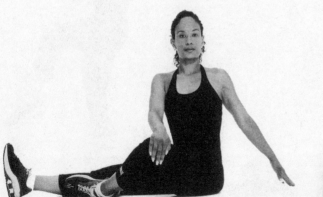

Figure 4.10

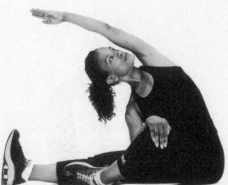

Figure 4.11

Piriformis Stretch

This is a good way to increase flexibility of the lower back muscles, particularly this often tight muscle.

1. Lie on your back and lift your right leg up, keeping your knee soft (not locked).

2. Put your left hand on your right knee and your right hand out to the side at chest level. (See Figure 4.12.)

3. Slowly rotate the right leg to your left side at the level of your belly button. (See Figure 4.13.)

4. Go only as far as you can without lifting your right shoulder off the floor.

5. Repeat four times.

6. Do same exercise with the left leg.

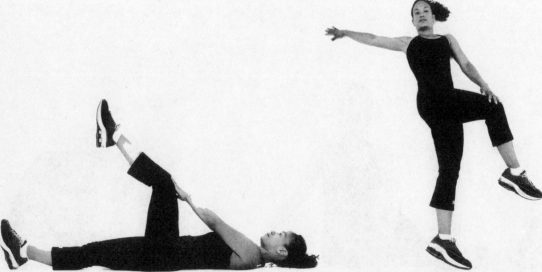

Figure 4.12

Figure 4.13

Back-Strengthening Exercises

Even if you have back pain, you should do these exercises. Use common sense in stopping if you feel sudden pain but don't be afraid to push yourself. Doing these will reap enormous rewards in increasing your strength and reducing or eliminating back pain.

Quadruped

This is a therapeutic exercise for people with chronic back pain. It is designed to strengthen the muscles that stabilize the spine.

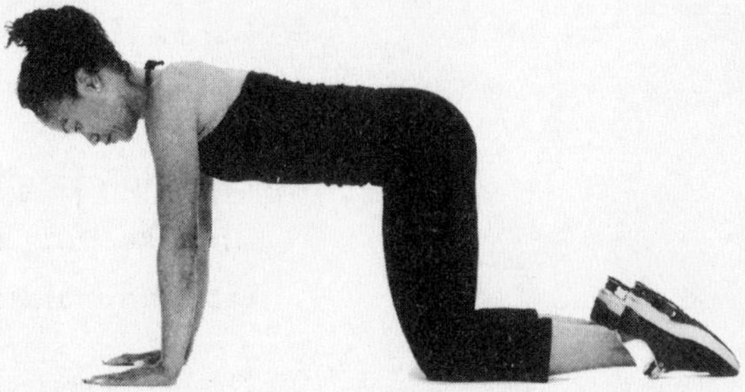

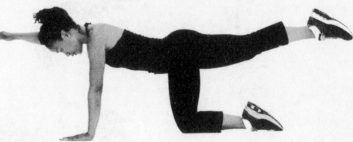

Figure 4.14

1. Get down on your hands and knees, arms directly below the shoulders and legs hip-width apart. Keep your back straight across like a table. (See Figure 4.14.)

2. Lift and straighten the right arm and left leg at the same time, keeping your shoulders down and away from your ears and maintaining your balance. (See Figure 4.15.)

3. Do three repetitions of 10 movements each.

4. Repeat exercise with opposite arm and leg.

Figure 4.15

IMPORTANT: Keep shoulders down. Also, if your hips are rocking from side to side it means you are having trouble with your balance. Keeping your stomach muscles tight will help you to stabilize your body.

Physio Ball Quadruped

This is the same quadruped exercise, using a physio ball to help you improve your balance by forcing you to stabilize your trunk on the ball while exercising

1. Lie on the physio ball, with the ball just under your chest. (See Figure 4.16.)

2. Lift and straighten the right arm and left leg at the same time, keeping your shoulders down and away from your ears and maintaining your balance. (See Figure 4.17.)

3. Do three repetitions of 10 movements each.

4. Repeat exercise with opposite arm and leg.

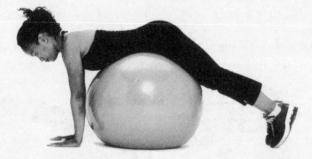

Figure 4.16

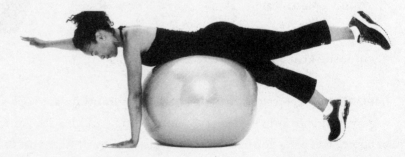

Figure 4.17

Prone Back Extension

This strengthens the muscles along the spine.

1. Lie on the floor, facedown, arms at your sides, legs straight out behind you. (See Figure 4.18.)

2. Keeping buttocks, legs, and stomach muscles tight, slowly lift your chest off the floor. (See Figure 4.19.)

3. Repeat 10 times.

IMPORTANT: Use back muscles, not arm muscles, to lift your chest.

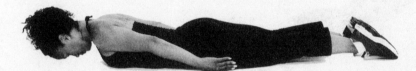

Figure 4.18

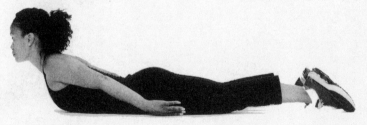

Figure 4.19

Back Extension on the Physio Ball

This exercise strengthens the muscles that stabilize your spine.

1. Lie on your stomach on the physio ball, arms at sides, legs together, hip-width apart, toes touching the floor. (See Figure 4.20.)

2. Holding your trunk still, lift your chest slowly. (See Figure 4.21.)

3. Squeeze your butt muscles, holding for five seconds.

4. Repeat 10 times.

IMPORTANT: Keep your shoulders down.

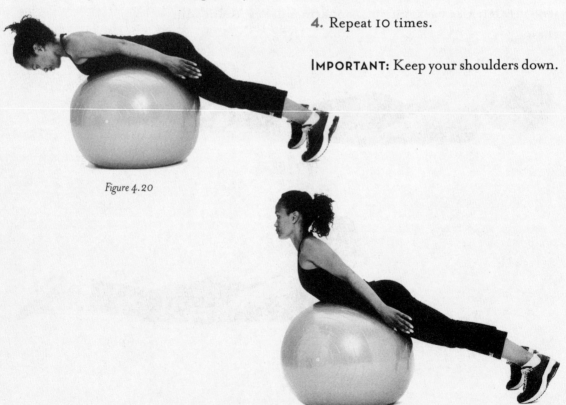

Figure 4.20

Figure 4.21

5

Why Hips Get
Out of Whack

When I shout, "Hip, hip, hooray!" I'm the one actually cheering for the hips. Hips are the largest and strongest joints in the body, responsible for bearing the weight of the upper body when you are standing and enabling you to move your lower body efficiently.

Because hips are so important in movement, when something goes wrong with them it is no small thing.

Some hip problems are out of your control, like traumatic injuries, congenital deformities and degenerative problems, all of which require a doctor's care.

But most people who suffer from hip pain are unwitting architects of their own discomfort. Poor body conditioning, weak and tight muscles, being overweight and not taking care of their bodies as they get older are the primary reasons for hip pain.

Usually these problems evolve over time so that you don't automatically make a connection between your activities and your hip pain.

As a result, you might be surprised to discover yourself in some of my clients who, with varying lifestyles, had all brought on their own hip pain. As we worked together, they were able to reduce or eliminate their pain and vastly improve how they looked and felt.

POOR BODY CONDITIONING

Diane, a woman in her early thirties, loves karate, not only because of its physical challenges but because she likes the discipline of working toward the belts you are awarded as you improve. She took classes two or three times a week for nearly a year, but then began to develop hip pain after her classes. The pain became so debilitating that she went to the doctor, who told her she had a groin pull and recommended that she take a rest from karate.

Loath to abandon her favorite activity, she came to me to learn some exercises to get rid of her pain without stopping her training. In our assessment I saw that, although Diane thought she was strong and fit from her sport, her outer hip muscles were very weak and her inner thigh muscles lacked flexibility. By repeatedly performing side kicks in class, she had aggravated her hip joint and overstretched her inner thigh muscles, which had led to small, extremely painful tears in the muscles. This is when the doctor told Diane she had a groin pull.

This injury is very common to physically active people who put great demands on their legs. Dancers, runners, soccer and basketball players all need strong and flexible hip muscles to perform efficiently and without injury.

When I explained this to Diane, she understood why the doctor had recommended she stop her sport while her muscles healed, and she was ready to begin a more comprehensive exercise program to stretch her inner thigh muscles and strengthen her outer hip muscles.

After a month of conscientious exercise, she was much stronger so that when she did return to her karate class, she had far more strength and was more flexible, and she easily passed the test for her yellow belt.

For Diane and other active people, it helps to understand that while the body is designed for movement, in fact thrives on movement, you have to meet it at least halfway by keeping it strong for what you want to do. It is very important to have a balance of strength, flexibility and endurance throughout your musculoskeletal system *before* you embark on a specific strenuous physical activity.

WEAK AND TIGHT MUSCLES

Alex is a slim young man in his twenties who relied on regular spinning classes to keep fit, and he looked great. However, he could hardly sleep because of hip pain when he lay in bed.

Alex took spinning classes up to four times a week, leaning forward over his bike and using the same muscles for an hour at a time as he furiously pedaled his way to fitness. Like many devotees of spinning, he assumed his high-intensity workout provided him with all the exercise he needed. And while spinning is great aerobic exercise, it's not a comprehensive workout for building strength and flexibility. In fact, by using the same hip muscles over and over, spinning puts stress on many of the components of the hip, creating imbalances in the muscles that stabilize the hips. Over time Alex's posture suffered, and his hip flexor muscles became very tight and stressed from overuse.

Eventually, this tightness created small tears in the strained tendons in front of the hip. The affected tendon swelled substantially and became very sensitive, painful enough to wake Alex at night when he rolled over onto his hip. This injury, called hip tendinitis, is very common in indoor and outdoor cyclists.

It took some time to convince Alex that he needed to prepare his body for his spinning sessions. Younger people like Alex, who is 24, tend to assume that their bodies will do anything asked of them with no problem and are often resistant to the idea of exercising for function rather than only aesthetics.

But one of the few good things about pain is that it forces you to pay attention, so when Alex understood that a comprehensive strength and stretching exercise program was the most effective way to relieve his pain, he signed on to my program.

Now he is much stronger, his posture has improved, and he's practically become a recruiter for me.

SEDENTARY AND OVERWEIGHT

Andy, in his early forties, was overweight and very sedentary in his habits. He was actually somewhat proud of the fact that he didn't buy into what he called the "fitness craze." Not for him carrying around bottled water, going to the gym, running in 10Ks, or taking up a sport. He did some walking, which he thought was plenty of exercise, but spent most of his time sitting either at his desk at work or in front of the television watching sports.

But in the months before he came to see me, he had begun to get severe pain in his hips whenever he stood for any period of time, like waiting beside his car while his gas tank filled up.

Why, he asked in desperation, do my hips hurt when I don't do anything to strain them?

The answer was that he was spending so much time in a seated position that his hip muscles had become shortened and tight. When he stood up, these tight muscles couldn't do their job of supporting his body, including his extra weight, and the ensuing pressure on the hips caused him considerable pain.

Because he had never done much exercise, Andy was extremely stiff and had very limited range of motion not only in his hips but throughout his body, so our early workouts consisted mainly of stretching exercises to ease the tightness in his muscles.

Gradually he began to feel better and was willing to begin an exercise program to improve his flexibility and posture. I told him it was also very important for him to begin a cardiovascular exercise program to help him lose weight. The many problems of overweight and obesity are very much in the news now, but Andy found his motivation to lose weight when he made the connection between his weight and the extra pressure he was putting on his hip joints.

Despite his disdain for exercise, Andy worked out with determination and very quickly began to lose weight and feel better. He claimed he was going to stop as soon as his hips stopped hurting, but he's been coming to the gym for almost six months. His posture has improved, he's lost some weight, is stronger, and looks much younger than he did when he first showed up in the gym. And his hips don't hurt anymore.

DEGENERATION DUE TO AGE

Robert was a retired ironworker in his late fifties who had terrible hip pain. Years of heavy lifting and constant hammering in his job had caused considerable wear and tear on his joints, and he was under a doctor's care for osteoarthritis. Walking for any distance was torture for him, and he was worried that he was heading for hip replacement surgery, which he did not want at all, so his doctor recommended that he begin an exercise program to strengthen and stretch his hip muscles.

While Robert's job had been particularly strenuous and hard on his hips, his overall condition was not that different from that of many people his age. As we get older, the cartilage that surrounds the hip joints begins to harden and get thinner so that it loses some of its protective capacity. Without the thicker cartilage helping the bones glide easily, movement becomes more difficult, even painful. The breakdown of this cartilage is osteoarthritis, and it can also lead to changes in the bones, which become more brittle and susceptible to fracture and breakage.

It is when this deterioration continues to the point where someone can no longer function in any way without severe pain that doctors recommend a total hip replacement.

The statistics on this are rather grim. According to the National Institute on Aging, half of people over sixty-five are affected by osteoarthritis, and more than 150,000 hip replacements are performed each year.

But cartilage degeneration can be significantly delayed if, along with a healthy diet, all the muscles of the hip area are kept strong and flexible and good posture is maintained.

I talked to Robert about this and explained to him that while we couldn't restore his cartilage and couldn't promise that he wouldn't need surgery, we could begin an exercise program to strengthen and stretch the muscles around his hip joint so that they could play a more active role in keeping the hip healthy and minimize the strain on his hip. This would reduce the pressure on the joint itself, lessening his pain when he moved. We would also do exercises to improve his posture, so that his alignment would improve, increasing the strength of the trunk and further relieving pressure on the hip joint.

Robert was very hesitant to exercise for fear of bringing on more pain, so we started very slowly with gentle stretching exercises and simple strengthening exercises until he began to enjoy some relief from his pain and realized I wasn't an agent of agony. He is now doing exercises that he never dreamed he would be able to do, his range of motion has improved significantly, and he is no longer in pain when he takes walks with his granddaughter.

WHAT'S YOUR HIP STORY?

If, like the clients I described, you have pain in your hips, you can begin to identify the source of the pain and exercise to reduce or eliminate your discomfort.

Even if you're pain-free, you could be heading for hip problems. If it's difficult for you to sit cross-legged on the floor in a relaxed way, if you walk tilted forward from the waist or if the heels of your shoes are worn down on either side rather than in the center, you could have very tight hip muscles, or imbalances in the strength of your hip muscles that could be affecting your gait and alignment.

It's important to pay attention to these often subtle signs of alignment problems because you can exercise your way back to hip health before you incur pain or injury.

WHY THE HIP NEEDS YOUR SUPPORT

The hip joint is the strongest in the body, supporting the weight of your upper body when you stand and move, bearing more than twice your body weight with each step you take and absorbing most of the stress of impact on your body when you're active. On top of this, of course, the hip allows you to move your legs in every direction. To do all this, the hip has more joints and muscles than any other part of the body, all working together in a dazzling symphony.

The hip joint is very strong, and people often take its many functions for granted. But learning how your hips work and how to exercise the muscles that surround them will reap large benefits, not only reducing your risk for injury, but enabling you to move with more strength and efficiency.

Bones and Joints and Cartilage

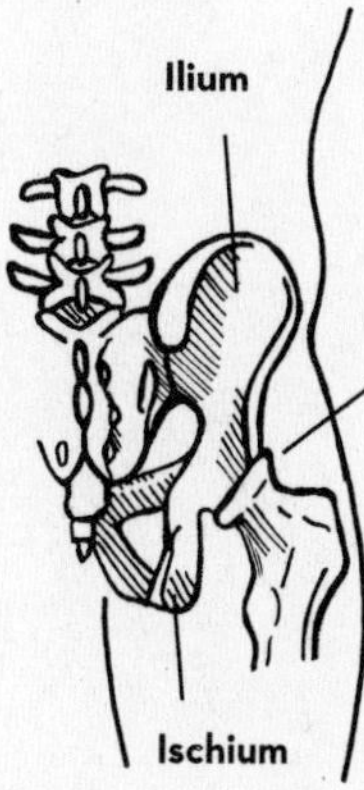

The hip is formed by the pelvis and the head of the thigh bone, called the femur. Three bones make up the pelvis: the ilium, the ischium, and the pubis. (See Figure 5.1.) Included in the hip are seven joints that allow you to move your spine, hips, and legs, including the sacroiliac joints, which facilitate movement where the hip and spine meet.

The stars of the hip, however, are the large hip joints that hold your thigh bones in place.

The acetabulofemoral joint is a large, deep ball-and-socket joint designed to hold your thigh bone in place and at the same time allow you to move your legs in any direction. (See Figure 5.2.) When kept strong and in alignment, the components of this joint work magnificently to stabilize your hip girdle while you perform your daily activities.

Cushioning the joint against the impact of your weight is a ring of cartilage that covers the head of the femur like a sleeve. Called the labrum, the cartilage increases the depth of the joint, providing additional sta-

Figure 5.1

Ilium

Acetabulo-
femoral
joint

Ischium

Figure 5.2

Hip joint with flexed hip

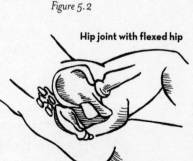

bility, smooths the way for movement, and prevents bone-on-bone contact between the femur and the pelvis.

The cartilage is quite vulnerable to injury, due to wear and tear caused by the stresses of weight-bearing movement on the joints and to natural degeneration as you age. These cause it to become thinner and worn. Exercise and proper alignment, however, can do a great deal to maintain its health and slow the degeneration process.

Ligaments

Ligaments connect bones to bones, and there are four in the hip joint—two in the front, one on the side, and one in the back. Like the cartilage, ligaments act as stabilizers to hold the joint in place and can become tense and stressed when imbalances in the muscles put pressure on the hip joint.

Of particular importance is the iliofemoral ligament, because it stabilizes the femur within the hip socket and helps to keep your hip girdle in a neutral position, which prevents sway-back. If the ligament is too tight, it compresses the femur in the hip joint, restricting mobility. If it's too loose, it causes hypermobility and instability of the femur when you move. Either of these conditions is a common cause for injury and pain among my clients.

Muscles

There are nearly three dozen muscles in your hips, all working together to give you the power to move your lower body. The difference in your movement when these muscles are strong compared to when they're not can be dramatic. My clients, even those who have been in pain, have far greater endurance after a few months of exercising and strengthening these muscles.

The structure of the hip joint allows you a wide range of movement and includes more muscles than you need to know about. But the summary below gives you an idea of the major muscle groups and what they do, as well as highlights some of the more common hip problems people face.

- Flexion is forward movement when you run or kick a ball, and there are nine flexor muscles that contribute to this action. One of these in particular, the iliopsoas, is a major postural muscle that needs to be strong to keep your bones in alignment. Often this muscle is weak and tight, and in combination with weak abdominals can create a *swayback*.

- Adduction brings the legs together, a movement enabled by five adductor muscles. *Groin pulls* are the result of one or several of these muscles being overstretched, causing very painful strains and tears in the muscles.

- Extension allows you to move your legs behind you. The gluteus maximus is the better known extensor muscle, along with some hamstring muscles, but a deep muscle called the piriformis is also very important in this movement. The piriformis (see Figure 5.3) lies over the sciatic nerve, and when it becomes tight, it presses down on the nerve, causing often severe pain. A doctor may diagnose this as *piriformis syndrome*.

- Abduction is when you open your legs, doing a jumping jack or a side kick. The primary

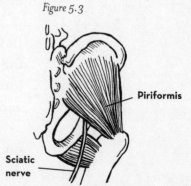

Figure 5.3

Piriformis

Sciatic nerve

muscles involved here are the two gluteal muscles, the gluteus minimus and the gluteus medius.

- Rotation is the ability to turn your legs in and out the way dancers do. There are nearly a dozen small muscles positioned very close to the hip joint that assist the femur in these movements and work to stabilize the hip joint.

Because of their proximity to the hip joint, it is important that the hip rotator muscles be strong to stabilize the hip. But usually they're not. Most people instead focus on exercising the larger muscles of the joint because they can see them and they want them to look good. But when these deep muscles are exercised, the risk of injury decreases significantly and movement becomes far more efficient.

Bursae and Tendons

Tendons connect muscles to bones and are dependent upon the strength of the muscles to which they're attached to maintain their health and flexibility. Weak and tight muscles can put unnecessary stress on tendons, causing them to swell and become inflamed, resulting in microscopic tears. This is when the doctor reports that you have *tendinitis*.

Between the tendons and the bones are bursae, small, fluid-filled sacs that act as cushions, reducing friction between the tendons and bones and absorbing the shocks placed on the joints during movement. There are several of them in the hip, and they are the front line of defense against pain.

Wear and tear on the hip, overuse, and tight muscles can cause bursae to become compressed and inflamed. This condition is *hip bursitis,* a common and painful hip injury.

RETURNING THE HIP TO HOME BASE

Understanding how your hip works and why it's important to keep the hip joint healthy can motivate you to exercise the muscles around your hip. Following are the exercises I give my clients to stretch and strengthen their hip muscles. Even if you don't suffer from hip pain, you can benefit mightily from including these exercises in your regular workouts.

Strengthening Exercises

There are often significant imbalances in the strength of the hip muscles that can lead to pain. These exercises will help you strengthen all your hip muscles equally.

Clams

This exercise strengthens the outer muscles of the hip, as strong hip muscles help keep the knee in its proper position.

1. Lie on your left side, with your elbow supporting your upper body. (If you have shoulder problems, lie down and support your head with your hand.)

2. Keeping your back straight, bend your knees and bring them forward so that your heels are under your hip. (See Figure 5.4.)

3. Lift your right leg up, keeping your knee bent. Rotate leg and knee up and back until your knee points toward the ceiling. Putting your hand on your hip helps to keep you from rolling your hips back as you rotate your leg. (See Figure 5.5.)

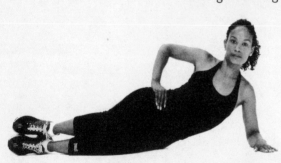

Figure 5.4

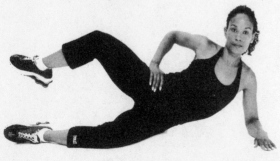

Figure 5.5

4. With your knee facing the ceiling, extend your leg back behind the hip. At the top of the movement, squeeze your outer hip and butt muscles. Lower your leg.

5. Do three sets of 15 repetitions.

6. Repeat exercise on the other side.

IMPORTANT: If your hips rotate back when you move your leg, it means you're pushing your leg out too far. Your hips need to remain stable to get the benefits of this exercise.

External Rotation with Abduction

This is an excellent exercise to strengthen the outer hip muscles, including the gluteus medius.

1. Lie on your left side, supporting your upper body with your elbow.

2. Bend your left leg back to help stabilize your body.

3. Keeping your right leg straight, turn your toe toward the floor. (See Figure 5.6.)

4. Lift the right leg up, rotating the toe outward toward the ceiling as you lift. (See Figure 5.7.)

5. Do three sets of 15 repetitions.

6. Repeat exercise with the left leg.

IMPORTANT: Don't roll your hips back as you move your leg. It helps to put your hand on your hip to remind you to keep your hips in alignment.

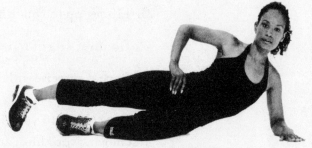

Figure 5.6

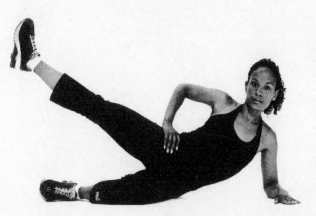

Figure 5.7

Diagonal Pattern

This is a good exercise for all the small muscles that stabilize the hip joint.

1. Lie on back, leaning back on your elbows, right leg straight out with toes turning inward, arms at your side. With foot flat on the floor, bend left knee. (See Figure 5.8.)

2. Lift your right leg up (see Figure 5.9) and out to the side (see Figure 5.10), rotating your foot outward as you lift.

3. Lift leg up to rotate back to start. (See Figure 5.11.)

4. Do three sets of 15 repetitions.

5. Repeat exercise with the left leg.

IMPORTANT: Lift your leg outward only as far as you can without moving your hips, and concentrate on using your core muscles to stabilize your hips.

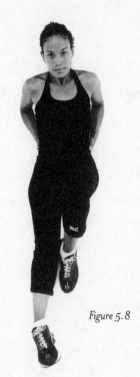

Figure 5.8

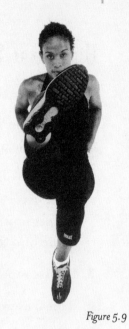

Figure 5.9

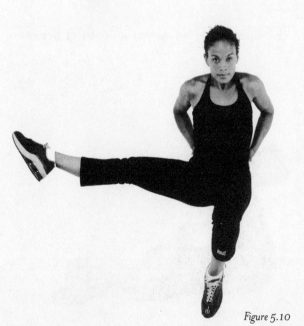

Figure 5.10

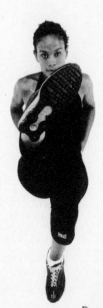

Figure 5.11

Hip Flexor Strengthener

This exercises the muscles that you use to move forward.

1. Lie on your back and bring your legs up so that your knees are at right angles to the floor.

2. Keeping your back flat on the floor—there should be no space between the back and the floor—push your hands against your left knee, feeling the contraction in the front of the hip. (See Figure 5.12.)

3. Do five repetitions, each time holding for a count of five.

4. Repeat exercise on your right knee.

IMPORTANT: Keep back flat on the floor and use your stomach muscles to help you with the exercise.

Progression: Do the same exercise pressing a towel between your knees.

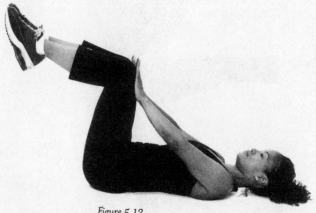

Figure 5.12

Stretching Exercises

These are wonderful stretching exercises if your hip muscles are stiff and sore. None of them should hurt, however. Stretch only as far as is comfortable.

Hip Flexor/Psoas Stretch

This is an important exercise to stretch these often tight muscles and return them to their normal resting lengths.

1. Kneel on one knee beside your bed or a physio ball, resting your arm on the bed or ball and keeping your other foot on the floor. (See Figure 5.13.)

2. Tuck your butt into a pelvic tilt and lean forward on the right leg, feeling the stretch in the front of the left thigh. (See Figure 5.14.)

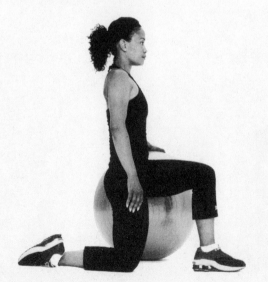

Figure 5.13

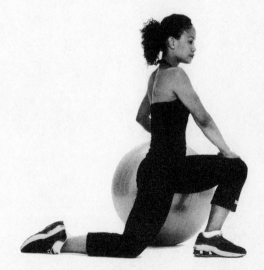

Figure 5.14

3. Hold for three seconds. Repeat up to eight times.

4. Switch legs and repeat exercise.

IMPORTANT: Maintain your pelvic tilt throughout the exercise so that you are isolating and stretching the hip flexor muscles.

Standing Outer Hip Stretch

This exercise releases tension in the outer hip, which can sometimes contribute to a tight iliotibial band described in chapter 6.

1. Stand next to a wall so that you can put your left arm at a right angle on the wall, elbow to hand resting against the wall.

2. Cross your right leg in front of your left leg at the ankle. (See Figure 5.15.)

3. Keeping your weight on your left leg, lean toward the wall so that you feel the stretch on the outside of your left hip. (See Figure 5.16.)

4. Hold for three seconds. Repeat up to eight times.

5. Repeat exercise on the opposite side.

IMPORTANT: Keep your butt in and stomach muscles tight.

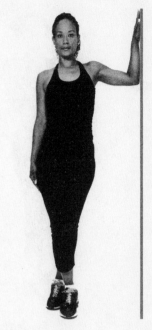

Figure 5.15

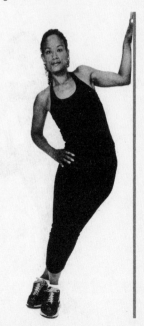

Figure 5.16

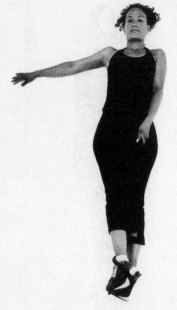

Figure 5.17

Outer Hip Stretch No. 2

You need a bathrobe tie or other rope for this exercise.

1. Wrap the rope around your right foot so that you can pull your foot toward you.

2. Lie on your back, making sure there is no space between your back and the floor. (See Figure 5.17.)

3. Keeping your stomach muscles tight and using the rope, slowly pull your leg across your body so you feel a full stretch on the outer hip. (See Figure 5.18.)

4. Hold for three seconds. Repeat up to eight times.

5. Repeat with the left leg.

IMPORTANT: Concentrate on keeping your back flat against the floor and your stomach muscles tight.

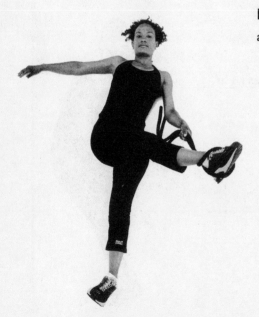

Figure 5.18

Inner Thigh and Groin Stretch

This is the same basic exercise using a rope, but it stretches the adductor muscles, which bring the legs together.

1. Wrap the rope around your right foot so that you can pull the foot outward away from your body.

2. Lie on your back, making sure there is no space between your back and the floor, right leg straight and left leg bent, and turn your right foot inward, as if you were pigeon-toed. (See Figure 5.19.)

3. Keeping your stomach muscles tight and using the rope, slowly pull your right leg away from your body. (See Figure 5.20.)

4. Repeat up to eight times.

5. Repeat with the left leg.

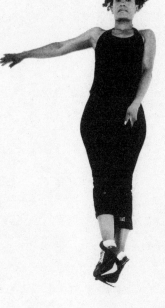

Figure 5.19

IMPORTANT: Concentrate on keeping your back flat against the floor and your stomach muscles tight.

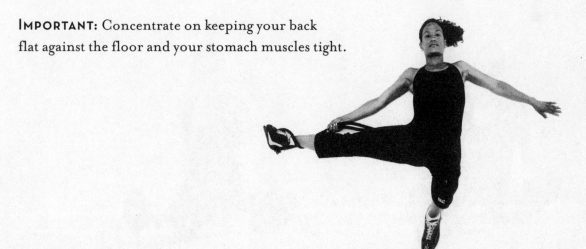

Figure 5.20

Seated Groin Stretch

This stretches the muscles in the front of your hips.

1. Sit on the floor, left leg straight, right leg bent at the knee, foot flat against the side of the left knee. (See Figure 5.21.)

2. Sit with good posture and gently lower your right knee as close as possible to the floor.

3. When you've gone as far as you can, gently press down on the right knee to feel a good stretch. (See Figure 5.22.)

4. Repeat up to eight times.

5. Repeat on the opposite leg.

IMPORTANT: Push your knee down only as far as you can without moving your back. Your back should remain neutral during this exercise.

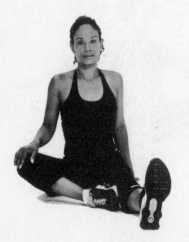

Figure 5.21

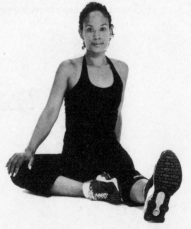

Figure 5.22

6

Why You Need
Your Knees

A lot of my clients tell me they have "bad knees," as if they're hobbling around on some kind of doomed stumps that will never bend and flex again. Nonsense. Most of the time a "bad" knee is just a "good" knee that needs attention.

However, things do seem to happen to knees more than to most other parts of the body. According to the American Academy of Orthopedic Surgeons, the most common reason people seek help from orthopedic surgeons is for knee pain.

If your knees bother you, answer the following questions:

- Are you overweight?

- Do you play tennis or squash, run regularly, or ski without doing any exercises to prepare yourself for your activity?

- If you do squats at the gym, do you bend too deeply in your squats?

- Do you have a predominantly sedentary lifestyle?

- Do you walk up stairs on the balls of your feet rather than planting your whole foot on the stair?

If the answer to any of these questions is yes, join the club. Being overweight, being either inactive or physically active without conditioning the body, poor exercise technique, and poor body mechanics are the most common reasons for knee problems that I see among my clients.

They aren't the only reasons, of course. Knees are quite vulnerable to injury, and many people have accidents that just happen—tears to the anterior cruciate ligament (ACL) are one example, as any skier can tell you. All the exercising in the world can't prevent freak accidents. Other people may have congenital abnormalities that increase their likelihood for knee pain.

But most of us can vastly improve the condition of our knees through targeted exercise and fitness training.

HOW KNEES GET KNOCKED AROUND

The fix-it to most knee problems, if they haven't progressed to the point where you need surgery, is to analyze your activities during the day so you understand how you use your knee and then to exercise the muscles that stabilize the knee to improve their strength and flexibility.

Strengthening and stretching the muscles that stabilize the knee joint also lowers the risk of knee accidents. Many people injure their knees during seemingly simple activities, and while you can't prevent all accidents, strong and flexible knee muscles combined with knowledge of the mechanics of the knee can reduce your risk for problems.

Finally, even if you've had surgery and physical therapy, you can prevent problems from recurring and often return your knees to full functionality by following an exercise program.

Below are the stories of a few of my clients who turned their knees around with functional exercises that increased the strength and flexibility of the muscles that stabilize their knees and greatly enhanced their performance.

JOY

I give Joy credit for showing up at the gym several months ago. In her thirties, she was quite overweight, not a common sight at the gym, and was self-conscious wearing her baggy sweats amid all the leotards and tank tops.

But her doctor had told her that the knee pain that she found so excruciating was due to the early stages of chondromalacia, which is a softening of the cartilage behind the kneecap.

Further, he told her the probable cause of the condition was her weight and the fact that she did little or no exercise. Lose twenty pounds and your knees will get better, he said, and so Joy had bravely signed up for a fitness session with me.

She complained of knee pain walking up and down stairs as well and when she stood for any length of time. Because of her pain, she had severely curtailed her activities. She'd even hired a dog walker to walk her dog because she was in so much pain.

I showed her, using an anatomy chart, how her extra weight, coupled with weak knee muscles, was putting great stress on her knee joint, compressing and stressing her bones and the ligaments and tendons surrounding them. This condition created episodes of terrible pain during her daily activities.

The good news, I told her, was that the doctor had said she hadn't yet caused any permanent damage to her knee, so that if she lost weight and began an exercise program she would significantly minimize the episodes of pain.

Asking people with knee pain to start an exercise program is tricky because putting weight on their knees, part of most cardiovascular exercise, is exactly what they can't do. But there are ways to get moving with minimal strain on the knees. At the gym, you can use elliptical machines, which allow you to walk and run without impact on your joints. Swimming and riding a stationary bike are also excellent aerobic exercises that are good for people like Joy because they provide a good cardiovascular workout without a weight-bearing component.

Along with a cardiovascular workout to help her lose weight, Joy and I worked on stretching and strengthening the muscles that stabilize her knees, which gave her immediate relief, so she could walk with less pain.

Exercising and stretching the muscles of her knees, along with gradual weight loss, have dramatically reduced Joy's knee pain and allowed her to become more active. She has more energy and feels a lot better about herself. It's nice to see her begin to live up to her name.

PETER

Peter, a young man who worked out four times a week, had a tear in his meniscus and was facing surgery. The doctor had sent him to me to strengthen the muscles around his knee joint before the surgery so his recovery time would be less.

Peter was very upset because he thought he was in great shape and didn't understand how he had gotten hurt.

But when he showed me how he did his squats, I knew. Many people who work out at the gym don't understand proper body mechanics and so don't know how to do exercises in a safe and efficient way. When you do squats, as Peter did, you should bend your knees no farther than a 90-degree angle so that your butt never goes below your knees, and your knees should never reach beyond the balls of your feet. Further, you need to distribute your weight equally between the ball of your foot and your heel when you are squatting.

But Peter was regularly doing very deep knee bends, so that

instead of strengthening the muscles around his knees, he was putting too much stress on his knee joints. On top of this, he was working out with heavy weights and putting most of his weight on the balls of his feet. All these things had irritated the cartilage in between his knee joint.

In addition, he never stretched his muscles to keep them flexible, nor did his workout include exercises to train all the muscles that help in stabilizing the knee. Over time, he had created tightness and imbalances in the muscles around the knee joint, which, added to the strains on the cartilage from improper exercise technique, had caused his meniscus to tear.

Peter was in a lot of pain, which is very common among those with knee problems. Knees can really hurt.

Our first goal was to alleviate some of his pain, which I did by showing Peter some stretches to help his muscles become more flexible and take stress off the knee joint. He became more comfortable right away.

At the same time we began a series of strengthening exercises for his muscles, not only the muscles that stabilize the hip and knee joints, but the muscles of his core. Strong core muscles support and enhance the movement of the muscles of the hip and knee, which is key to efficient joint movement. Peter found that this more comprehensive workout was much more effective and dramatically reduced the strain on his knee.

Along with his new workout, I explained some basic anatomy to Peter so that he understood how his knee worked, and how important it is to use proper technique when exercising. We went over all his exercises carefully so he would continue his workouts safely.

Peter's surgery to clean out the loose cartilage in his knee was a success and he now is back at the gym, delighted to be pain-free and much more knowledgeable about how to stay that way.

JEFF

Jeff was another refugee from the doctor's office, where he had been diagnosed with strained ligaments from running and told to stop the sport.

Hardly willing to give up an activity he had enjoyed for many years, Jeff, a fit man in his mid-forties, decided to start fitness training in hopes of improving his strength and flexibility.

I see many clients like Jeff who have been physically active for their whole lives but do no conditioning for the sports they enjoy. Runners, particularly, assume that because they run their legs are strong and they don't have to do any other lower body exercise. This isn't true. Running does not provide a complete workout for the muscles of the hips and knees. In fact most runners' injuries are created by their lack of overall conditioning for their sport.

Jeff was no exception. Other than a few quick stretches, he did no preparation before he ran, so his muscles were very tight. In addition, while some of his hip and knee muscles were strong, others were very weak, and the result of these imbalances in conjunction with the repetitive motion of running had put undue pressure on the ligaments of his knee. The result was that he had a burning pain on the outer part of his knee every time he ran.

I explained to him that a good functional exercise program that strengthened all the muscles of the hip and knee would ease the strain on his ligaments so he could eventually resume running without pain.

Also important for Jeff was to really stretch his muscles both before and after exercise. Stretching keeps the muscles flexible and the joints healthy.

Humbled by his aching knees, Jeff began the program I designed, and reported an immediate relief from his pain. As his muscles became stronger and more flexible, he was able to resume his running and no longer suffered from the burning bouts of pain that had sidelined him.

KNOW YOUR KNEE

If you think about all the ways you use your knees throughout the day, from simply walking from point A to point B to practically any kind of exercise, you'll realize the tremendous strain you are putting on your hip and knee joints. Every time you take a step, all your weight comes to bear through the joints of the hip and knee. Multiply that weight tenfold when you jump or run. If you add to that the pressures on the knee joint from the problems described above, it's no surprise that orthopedists see so many knee patients.

Want to know why your knees are aching? The first step is to learn how they work.

Knee Joint

The knee is a hinge joint. It moves your lower leg back and forth when you walk, run, and kick. The joint is not built to rotate clockwise or counterclockwise, and it can be quite vulnerable to injury. Skiers, football players, and soccer players who have popped their anterior cruciate ligament (ACL) know this too well.

Knee Bones, Cartilage, and the Iliotibial Band

There are four bones that create the knee: the thigh bone, or femur; the lower leg bones, called the tibia and the fibula; and the kneecap, called the patella.

The bones are covered by articular cartilage—tough, smooth fibrous tissue that caps the bone and eases the joint movement. Between the bones are two pads of cartilage, called menisci, which prevent bone-on-bone contact and act as shock absorbers when you put weight on the joint. This cartilage also helps stabilize the joint. (See Figure 6.1.)

The iliotibial band is a thick band of tissue that runs from the middle of the femur, down the outside of the thigh to just below the knee joint. It acts as a stabilizer when you run, but when this band gets tight, as often happens, it can create problems in the alignment of the kneecap. (See Figure 6.2.)

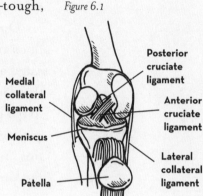

Figure 6.1

Posterior cruciate ligament

Medial collateral ligament

Anterior cruciate ligament

Meniscus

Lateral collateral ligament

Patella

Muscles

Many people think there are only two muscles around the knee—one hamstring muscle and one quadriceps muscle. Think again! There are nearly a dozen muscles that surround your knee that are equally important in keeping your knee joint in alignment and functioning properly. Once you know they're there, and understand how much they will improve the strength of your knee joint, you can easily exercise them all in your workouts.

The knee muscles come in two groups: the flexors, which allow you to lift your foot off the floor, and the extensors, which you use to straighten your legs.

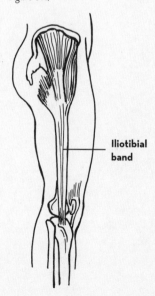

Figure 6.2

Iliotibial band

Among the flexors, there are three hamstring muscles behind the knee, semimembranosus, the semitendinosus, and biceps femoris. Three more secondary flexor muscles are the muscles in your calf, the popliteus, gastrocnemius, and soleus. If you keep them strong and flexible, they contribute to the efficiency and stability of the knee joint.

Opposing the flexors so that you can return your foot to the floor are the extensor muscles, called quadriceps, which are located at the front and sides of your knee. Important among them is the vastis medialus oblique (VMO), which is attached to the patella near the inside of the knee. If you put your fingers next to your kneecap on the inside of your leg, you can feel this muscle when you extend your leg. All the muscles around the knee work together to keep the kneecap in place when you flex and extend your leg.

One of the biggest problems I see is that the muscles that attach at the knee become very weak and tight, creating a lot of tension on the ligaments and tendons of the knee joint and alignment problems of the kneecap. Also very common is that people exercise some of the knee muscles but not others, which creates imbalances in muscle strength and increases the risk for knee dysfunction. Clients know lots of exercises to strengthen their quadriceps, for instance, but haven't even heard of the VMO, let alone exercise this important muscle.

Because of this lack of knowledge about knee anatomy and not understanding the importance of total knee exercise, people needlessly increase their risk for pain and injury in the knees. At the end of this chapter are exercises to stretch the muscles around the knee as well as ways to exercise all the muscles equally.

Knee Ligaments

The ligaments are key players in the knees, and, boy, do they have their work cut out for them. There are four of them, and they have to stabilize the knee joint against any extreme movement in any direction, a tough job when people are physically active. The ligaments, as a result, are the most common site for knee injuries.

Connecting and stabilizing the tibia and femur on the outside of your knee is the lateral collateral ligament (LCL); doing the same job on the inside of the knee is the medial collateral ligament (MCL).

Deep inside the knee is the most notorious ligament, the anterior cruciate ligament (ACL). This long, thin ligament attaches the femur and tibia in their centers, and its job is to limit rotation and twisting of the knee joint as well as to restrain forward movement of the knee so that your tibia doesn't move beyond the femur. The ACL is actually very strong, but when the knee is forced into an extreme rotation, as happens in an accident during active sports, it can do only so much. It's no wonder that ACL tears and sometimes complete rips of the ligaments are so common among athletes.

The posterior cruciate ligament (PLC) is behind the knee, providing stability to the joint and limiting the backward movement of the tibia in relation to the femur.

Tendons, Bursae

The knee joint is also served by many tendons, which connect the muscles to the bones, and by bursae, fluid-filled sacs that act as shock absorbers in the knee joint. Unfortunately, when there are imbalances in knee muscles, the tendons and bursae feel the pressure and are often overstretched or compressed.

BAD THINGS THAT HAPPEN TO KNEES

There are as many types of injuries to the knee as there are muscles, ligaments, and tendons therein, and I'm not in the business of diagnosing knee complaints. But when you're learning about your knees, it's helpful to have an idea of what has gone wrong in your knee when the doctor tells you that you have an injury. Below are some of the more common knee injuries I see among my clients.

Osteoarthritis of the Knee

Osteoarthritis is a painful degenerative disease caused by the wearing down of the cartilage that protects the knee joint. As we age, our cartilage thins, narrowing the space between the bones and compressing the ligaments and tendons that support and surround the bones and muscles. These tissues become inflamed and swollen, often causing tremendous pain. While some degeneration is inevitable as we age, being overweight or physically inactive without being in good alignment can speed up the process.

Osteoarthritis affects more than 20 million Americans, mostly over the age of 45, according to the Arthritis Foundation, but its onset can be delayed if you keep the muscles of the knee strong and flexible so that the knee works efficiently.

Meniscal Tears

The menisci are two pads of cartilage that lie between the femur and the tibia, both stabilizing the bones and protecting them from bone-on-bone contact during movement. They are like small shock absorbers. When there is excessive weight coupled with poor body mechanics, usually because of tightness and strength imbalances in the muscles of the knee, the menisci can become compressed and strained. If this stress continues, even the slightest bit of rotation can cause a tear in the menisci, releasing meniscal fibers that float in the knee joint. When this happens you sometimes hear a click in the knee area when bending or straightening, or experience inflammation at the site. This is extremely painful and can require surgery to clean out the debris in the knee.

Chondromalacia

This is another cartilage-related knee injury that occurs when the cartilage behind the kneecap softens so much that the patella grinds against the femur and tibia when you move. As you can imagine, this really hurts. Common causes of chondromalacia, which can happen at any age, are being overweight or having weaknesses in the muscles of the knee, which create poor alignment of the knee. This results in pain when you use the knee, especially walking up and down stairs. Losing weight and exercise can significantly delay the progression of this condition.

Ligament and Iliotibial Band Strains

When you have pain and swelling on the inner or outer part of your knee, the doctor may report that you're suffering from ligament strains. These strains most often occur in people who are active in sports that require a lot of repetitive movement but who aren't in good physical condition for the activities they pursue. The ligaments in the knee are designed to keep the knee from excessive rotation, but when there is overuse of some muscles and under-use of others, imbalances are created in the strength of the muscles that surround and support the knee. The ligaments are then forced to take on more than their fair share of the stress of the movement during pivoting and rotation, and become strained. This very painful condition can be eased by a good exercise program.

The iliotibial band can be another source of knee pain. When the muscles surrounding the hip and knee are weak and tight, the iliotibial band can also become tight and may experience friction from rubbing against the tibia. This is an overuse injury that is very common to runners. The resulting pain—a sharp, burning sensation—can be alleviated by strengthening and stretching the outer muscles that surround the hip and knee.

ACL Tears

Tears in the ACL (anterior cruciate ligament) usually result from a forceful rotation of the knee while the foot remains firmly planted on the ground. If the tear is minor, strengthening of the muscles around the knee can sometimes enable a person to function without surgery. When subject to excessive torque, however, the ACL can rip completely, requiring immediate surgery.

This is an extremely common accident for skiers, whose feet and ankles are held in place and supported by ski boots. When they take a sudden turn, or fall down, their ski boots remain in one position, putting all the strain of the sudden rotation on their knee joint, and the ACL simply snaps from the strain.

Tendinitis and Bursitis

When the muscles of the knee are tight, weak, and out of alignment, the tendons that attach the muscles to the bones can become inflamed as they are forced to bear the strains of the weak muscles. Tendinitis is the result.

Similarly, the bursae, small, fluid-filled sacs positioned to act as cushions within the knee joint, can become compressed when the knee muscles are out of alignment. This painful condition is called bursitis.

Strengthening and stretching can improve the alignment of the muscles of the knee joint and can go a long way in reducing the pain of tendinitis and bursitis.

KNEE EXERCISES

Following are a number of stretching and strengthening exercises that will help alleviate knee pain you might be experiencing, as well as improve the flexibility and strength of all your knee muscles so that your knee joint can work efficiently and remain healthy.

Strengthening Exercises

These exercises will strengthen all the muscles that surround and protect your knee joints, decreasing your risk of injury. Anyone with knee problems should do these every day, as should weekend athletes who want to lower their risk for injury.

Leg Extension with Adduction

This exercise strengthens the inner thighs, the VMO, and the lower fibers of the quadriceps.

1. Sit in a chair, feet flat on the floor, and place a rolled towel or soft children's ball between your knees. Squeeze your knees together against the towel or ball. (See Figure 6.3.)

2. Extend your left leg straight out. (See Figure 6.4.) Bend the knee slowly, lowering the foot to the floor.

3. Do three sets of 20 repetitions.

4. Repeat the exercise with your right leg.

Progression: As you become stronger, you can add ankle weights to increase the benefits of this exercise. Start with two pounds and increase.

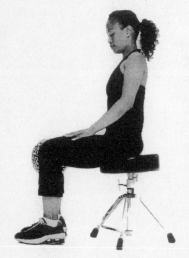

Figure 6.3

IMPORTANT: Keep squeezing your knees together against the towel or ball as you work. This exercise can also be done in the gym with the leg extension machine.

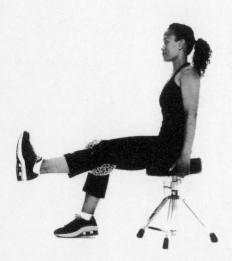

Figure 6.4

Step Ups

This is another way to strengthen the muscles that extend your knee.

1. Stand with your left foot on a step, footstool, or telephone book at about a 4-inch height. (See Figure 6.5.) Distribute your weight evenly between the ball and heel of your foot.

2. Step up on the stair on your left leg, keeping your stomach muscles tight and your weight forward on the working leg. Maintain good posture. (See Figure 6.6.)

3. Lower your body back down to the starting position.

4. Do two sets of 20 repetitions.

5. Repeat exercise with the right foot.

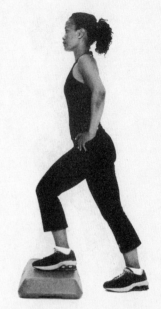

Figure 6.5

Progression: As you get stronger, you can do this exercise holding weights, starting with two pounds and increasing.

IMPORTANT: Concentrate on maintaining good posture and keeping your weight forward on the working leg. Using your stomach muscles will help you keep your balance.

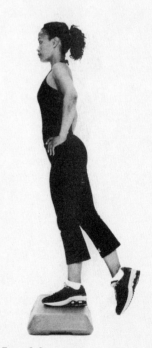

Figure 6.6

Step Downs

This will strengthen the leg muscles that help to bend, or flex, the knee.

1. Stand with both legs on a step, footstool or telephone book at about a 4-inch height.

2. Extend your right foot in front, only to help you maintain your balance. All your weight should be on the left foot. (See Figure 6.7.)

3. Keeping your weight on your left foot, bend your knees and hips as if you're going to sit down. Stand up, maintaining good posture. (See Figure 6.8.)

4. Do three sets of 20 repetitions.

5. Repeat exercise with the right leg.

Progression: As you get stronger, you can do this exercise holding weights, starting with two pounds and increasing.

IMPORTANT: Don't tuck your butt under, and concentrate on using your stomach muscles to help you maintain balance and keep good posture.

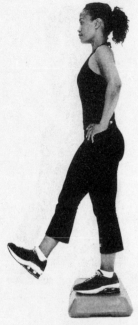

Figure 6.7

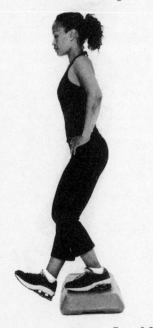

Figure 6.8

Knee Extension

This exercise strengthens the muscles that keep the knee in good alignment.

1. Tie a Thera-Band elastic band (green or blue strength) around a table leg, or some other object strong enough to withstand your weight pulling against it. The Thera-Band should be at knee height.

2. Slip the Thera-Band behind your left knee and stand far enough back to create tension. (See Figure 6.9.)

3. Bend the knee and squeeze your quadriceps, then straighten the leg. Keep your heel on the floor. (See Figure 6.10.)

4. Do two sets of 20 repetitions.

5. Repeat exercise with the right knee.

IMPORTANT: The Thera-Band must be at knee height for this exercise to work.

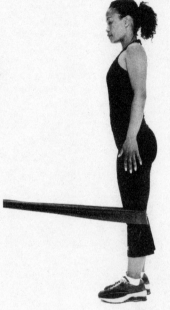

Figure 6.9

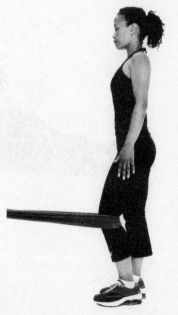

Figure 6.10

Clams

This is a hip exercise that is equally important for the knees, as strong hip muscles help support the function of the knee.

1. Lie on your left side, elbow supporting your upper body. (If you have shoulder problems, lie down and support your head with your hand.)

2. Keeping your back straight, bend your knees and bring them forward so that your heels are under your hip. (See Figure 6.11.)

3. Lift your right leg up, keeping your knee bent. Rotate leg and knee up and back until your knee points toward the ceiling. Putting your hand on your hip helps keep you from rolling your hips back as you rotate your leg. (See Figure 6.12.)

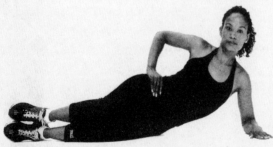

Figure 6.11

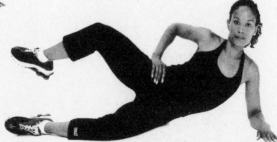

Figure 6.12

4. With your knee facing the ceiling, extend your leg back behind the hip. At the top of the movement, squeeze your outer hip and butt muscles. Lower your leg.

5. Do three sets of 15 repetitions.

6. Repeat exercise on the other side.

IMPORTANT: If your hips rotate back when you move your leg, it means you're pushing your leg out too far. Your hips need to remain stable to get the benefits of this exercise.

Leg Curl with Physio Ball

This exercise strengthens the muscles that help to flex the knee.

1. Lie on your back, legs straight, heels resting on the physio ball.

2. Lift hips off the floor. (See Figure 6.13.)

3. Keeping hips off the floor, bend knees and, using your heels, pull the physio ball toward you. (See Figure 6.14.)

4. Still keeping hips aloft, push ball away from you with your heels.

5. Do three sets of 15 repetitions.

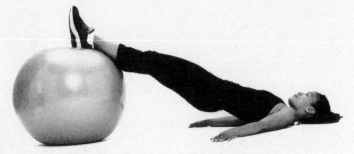

Figure 6.13

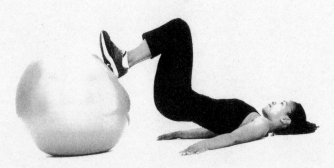

Figure 6.14

Stretching Exercises

These exercises will reduce the tension in your knee muscles and increase your flexibility and strength. You should do them before and after exercise. These exercises should not hurt, so modify the stretch if you feel pain. Over time your flexibility will increase and you will be able to increase your range of motion. Don't rush it.

Quadriceps Stretch

This exercise helps reduce tension in the knees.

1. Lie on the floor on your left side, with your knees at a 90-degree angle to your trunk.

2. Put your right hand on your right foot and place a rope around your left foot to hold the knee in place and stabilize the hip. (See figure 6.15.)

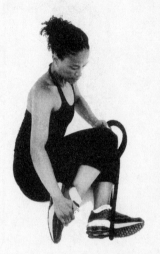

Figure 6.15

3. Keeping your left leg bent and contracting your glutes, pull your right knee back until it is directly under the hip. (See Figure 6.16.) Hold for three seconds and relax.

4. Repeat eight to ten times until you feel the release in the muscle.

5. Lie on the floor on your left side and repeat the exercise with your right leg.

IMPORTANT: If your muscles are very tight and this stretch causes pain, do the exercise with your lower leg straight instead of bent. Eventually your muscles will return to their normal resting length and your flexibility will increase.

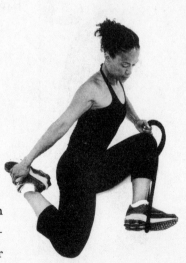

Figure 6.16

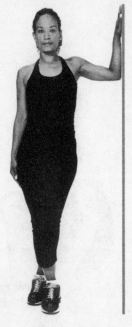

Figure 6.17

Standing Outer Hip Stretch

This exercise, also in the hip chapter, releases tension in the outer hip, which can sometimes contribute to a tight iliotibial band.

1. Stand next to a wall so that you can put your left elbow on the wall, elbow to hand resting against the wall.

2. Cross your right foot in front of your left foot at the ankle. (See Figure 6.17.)

3. Keeping your weight on your left leg, lean toward the wall so that you feel the stretch on the outside of your left hip. (See Figure 6.18.)

4. Repeat up to eight times.

5. Repeat exercise on the opposite side.

IMPORTANT: Keep your butt in and stomach muscles tight.

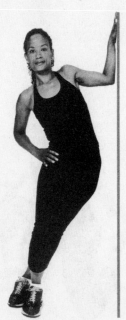

Figure 6.18

Heel Cord Stretch, Part 1

Many people don't know how to correctly stretch their calf muscles. This exercise does this and is excellent for runners both before and after running.

1. Sit on the floor, legs straight out in front of you, feet flexed, right foot on top of left foot, heel to toe. Put a towel or rope around your right foot. (See Figure 6.19.)

2. Keeping your back straight and maintaining good posture, lean forward over your leg. Flex foot and, squeezing the muscles around your kneecap, pull your toes toward you with the towel. (See Figure 6.20.)

3. Hold for three seconds. Repeat eight to ten times until you feel a release.

4. Reverse position so that your left foot is on top of your right foot and repeat the exercise.

IMPORTANT: Keep your back straight. Look for comfortable tension with this exercise, and ease up if you feel pain.

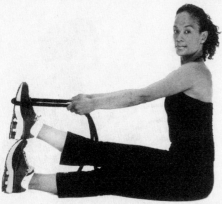

Figure 6.19

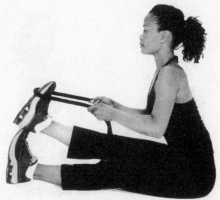

Figure 6.20

Heel Cord Stretch, Part 2

This exercise stretches your outer calf muscles.

1. Sit on the floor, legs straight out in front of you, feet flexed, right foot on top of left foot, heel to toe.

2. Put a towel or rope around your right foot. (See Figure 6.21.)

3. Rotate your right toe inward, as if you were pigeon-toed. Keeping your back straight and maintaining good posture, lean forward over the leg and, keeping toes flexed and facing inward and squeezing the muscles around your kneecap, pull your toes toward you with the towel. (See Figure 6.22.)

4. Hold for three seconds. Repeat eight to ten times until you feel a release.

5. Repeat exercise with the left foot.

IMPORTANT: Keep your back straight. Look for comfortable tension with this exercise, and ease up if you feel pain.

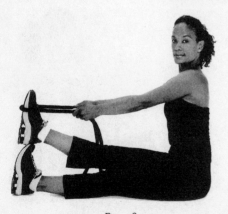

Figure 6.21

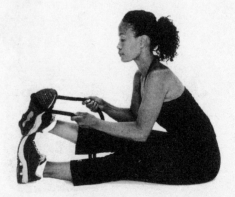

Figure 6.22

7

Shoulders and Neck—Loosen Up!

Typical of my clients in work-obsessed New York City is a 30-year-old woman named Claire. Working long hours and unable to keep up her running schedule, she wanted to get back in shape. She asked me to teach her how to use the machines at the gym to tone her stomach, arms, and legs so she could look like she did in college when she'd been an athlete. But the first thing I noticed about her wasn't what she noticed about herself—a general lack of muscle tone. Her posture was poor. Her shoulders were rounded forward and her head, instead of sitting properly on her shoulders, was leaning slightly forward. Her shoulders were lifted up around her neck, and she looked tired and stressed, and older than she was.

I knew that she probably worked at a desk all day, either leaning over a computer or talking on the telephone. Leaning forward in the same position day after day, Claire had slowly overstretched the muscles along her back, causing her shoulders to round forward. At the same time her chest muscles became shorter and tighter. The resulting imbalance made it difficult for her upper back muscles to assist in supporting her head and neck, so her head leaned forward.

I see this all the time. Office work can lead to terrible posture, one of the most common maladies I find among my clients. It is also one of the most aging. A little extra weight and thicker thighs don't affect how people look nearly as much as how they carry themselves.

But Claire didn't know this. Like so many young and generally fit people, she had never thought about the effect of her daily work routine on her body. She knew she wasn't as physically active as she should be, but she had no idea that she was sabotaging her body every day by sitting in one position all day.

I began to work with her to strengthen her weak shoulder muscles and improve her posture. By standing straighter she looked taller, thinner, and more confident and energetic. She told me that friends were asking her what she'd done, whether she'd cut her hair or lost weight. They thought she looked great. And she did. Improving her posture had restored her to the look she'd had in college.

As important, she learned that good posture improved not only her looks but her alignment as well. Her program minimized the stress on her muscles and significantly reduced her risk of shoulder injury.

SHRUGGING OFF BAD HABITS

There are a lot of people like Claire who have no idea that they have poor posture. Even if they are aware their shoulders aren't where they should be, they often don't think it matters.

But shoulder misalignment does matter. When the shoulder joint is not functioning properly, it can affect your range of motion. Further, shoulder misalignment can lead to stiffness and strains on the shoulder joint, and eventually to pain and injury. By exercising all the muscles of the shoulder girdle, however, you will greatly increase the strength of these muscles and their ability to stabilize the shoulder joint, correcting any imbalances and improving your shoulder function.

Whether you simply have poor posture, like Claire, or are

now experiencing some kind of neck or shoulder pain, it's worth your while to think about how you use your shoulders in your daily activities so you can identify whether you're bringing your shoulder problems on yourself. Below are some of the most common examples of daily activities that can lead to shoulder trouble.

Repetitive Movements

If you use the same shoulder muscles in the same way day after day, week after week, you are going to create imbalances, with certain muscles working overtime and others barely working at all.

When these imbalances in muscle strength become pronounced, your range of motion in your shoulders and arms can become limited. The imbalances also contribute to poor posture, which puts stresses on your muscles as well as other components of the shoulder and makes them vulnerable to injury.

The demands of desk work are probably the most common source of repetitive movement. If you're bending forward over your desk for hours at a time without taking a break, cradling the phone between your neck and shoulder rather than using a headset or rotating your body toward your computer, you could be creating shoulder dysfunction and poor posture.

Many activities, however, put strains on the shoulder and neck. A violinist who practices for five hours every day, holding her instrument on the same shoulder, moving the bow across her chest in the same direction, is just as much at risk for overuse of her shoulder and neck muscles as a computer programmer sitting at his desk.

Hairdressers spend a good part of their days holding their arms at shoulder level or higher while blow-drying clients' hair, making them vulnerable to pain and injury. A motorcyclist can suffer from strains on his neck and shoulders when the handles of his bike are either too low or too high.

Think about how you use your shoulder and neck muscles. What routine tasks do you do every day that involve your shoulders and neck? Do you neglect doing exercises to prepare your body for these daily activities? Do any of your shoulder activities cause you pain? If so, your movements might be affecting your posture and the range of motion of your shoulders, and you could be increasing your risk for an overuse injury.

Tension

I used to tease my college roommate Gwen that I knew when exams were coming by how she hunched her shoulders up toward her ears. People have their own way of holding stress, and Gwen always tensed her shoulders when she was under pressure at school.

Holding tension in your shoulders creates tightness in the muscles of the neck, so if you've dropped your shoulders while reading this, you've just released that tension.

Poor Training Techniques at the Gym

This is a surprisingly common source of shoulder and neck misalignment among those who work out regularly. At the gym you see a lot of men whose biceps and shoulder muscles are impressively big and well defined so that they look very fit. But when I work with them, I find that their muscles are extremely tight, and that they don't have normal range of motion in their neck and shoulders. This is usually because they work out with extremely heavy weights to build bulk and create definition in their larger, most visible muscles, but often neglect to strengthen the deeper muscles of the shoulder girdle. These deeper muscles support the shoulder joint and need to be trained along with the larger muscles to maintain good alignment of the shoulder joint, so you can enjoy the full range of motion in your shoulder.

Another common problem with bodybuilders is that they do little or no stretching, which creates tightness and inflexibility in the shoulder muscles.

But it's not just bodybuilders who need instruction in proper exercise technique. Everyone interested in general fitness would benefit from reviewing the way they work out. Do you choose the right exercises for your needs, exercises that are tailored to your own activities and that will enhance your fitness and prevent injury? Are you doing the exercises correctly?

One of the most common mistakes I see both men and women make at the gym, for instance, is to drop their elbows too low when doing chest presses. When you lie on your back on a bench holding weights, your elbows should never drop below your shoulder joints. Doing so compromises the integrity of tendons and ligaments in the shoulder, so that instead of strengthening your pectorals, you're creating potential problems in your shoulder joints.

Miscellaneous Everyday Habits

We all have habits that conspire against our posture, and if you think about your own, you might find that some are creating imbalances in your shoulder and neck muscles.

- Do you regularly carry a pocketbook, briefcase, computer, or schoolbag on one shoulder?

- When you are sitting down at work, in front of the television or at the dinner table, do you sit slumped in your chair?

- If you are large-breasted, do you tend to round your shoulders forward to deflect attention from your chest?

If you see yourself in any of these problems, you can begin a simple exercise program to correct the muscle imbalances you have created so that you will look and feel better. Your posture will improve and you will be able to conduct your regular activities with renewed efficiency and strength.

Before you go straight to the exercises at the end of this chapter, you could benefit from learning a little bit about the anatomy of your shoulder. This will help you understand why you need to exercise the muscles that surround your shoulder joint and how to do so correctly. Plus, my clients tell me it's fun to know what's going on in there.

THE SCOOP ON THE SHOULDER

If ever a body part should write to Ann Landers, complaining that it's misunderstood, it would be the shoulder. Here you have the most generous joint in the body, allowing you to swing your arm in any direction you want, and a wonderful set of muscles that help stabilize your head, neck, and shoulders and keep them in proper alignment.

However, not only do people not appreciate its versatility, they have no idea how the shoulder works or how important (and simple) it is to take care of it so it will serve you well.

Bones and Joints

Your shoulder consists of several large bones: the shoulder bone, which is called the scapula; the collarbone, called the clavicle, and the arm bone, called the humerus. Together they create the shoulder joint, called the glenohumeral joint.

This large ball-and-socket joint has the widest range of motion of any joint in the body, allowing you to move your hand in any direction. Lining it is cartilage, the glenoid labrum, which enhances the depth of the joint, helps stabilize it, prevents bone-on-bone contact in the joint, and reduces shock to the joint when you move. (See Figure 7.1.)

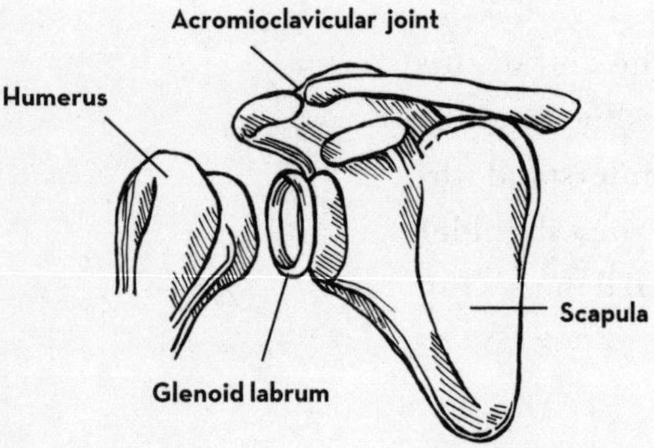

In order to allow you the full range of motion it does, the shoulder joint is very shallow. When you cup your palm over your computer mouse, your hand is sitting at about the same depth as the humerus sits in the joint.

Figure 7.1

Acromioclavicular joint

Humerus

Glenoid labrum

Scapula

The glenohumeral joint doesn't work alone, however. There are several other, smaller joints in the front, side, and back of the shoulder as well, all of which work together to create the dynamic for you to be able to move your hand. The acromioclavicular joint maintains the connection between the scapula and the collarbone; the sternoclavicular joint connects the collarbone to the sternum, and the scapular thoracic joint connects the shoulder to the upper back.

When you have good posture and are strong, these joints work well, but if you suffer from muscle tightness and/or poor posture, stresses can occur on the joints and the ligaments, tendons, and bursae surrounding them, leading to pain and injury.

Muscles

The shallowness of the glenohumeral joint combined with the mechanics of the other smaller shoulder joints makes it important that all shoulder muscles surrounding the joints be strong and flexible enough to stabilize and protect them.

The shoulder has two sets of muscles that work together to do this. The superficial, or large, muscles that are visible to the eye, allow you to navigate your hand through space. Beneath them are the deep muscles that are attached to your bones. These muscles stabilize and protect the shoulder joint, keeping the humerus in its proper position so the larger muscles have a stable base from which to move.

Superficial Muscles

Because you can see them, most people are familiar with the superficial muscles, like their lats, the latissimus muscles, and pecs, the pectoral muscles. These are the muscles we most often exercise, because we want them to look good.

The primary superficial muscles in addition to the lats and pecs are the deltoids and the large trapezius muscles.

Figure 7.2

There are three deltoid muscles surrounding the scapula that give shape to your shoulders and allow you to lift your arms up and away from your body. The pectoral muscle, called the pectoralis major (see Figure 7.2), is an elongated muscle that runs across either side of your chest. You use them when you're pushing a door open. When you want to close a door, you use your latissimus dorsi, which are wide muscles that cover both sides of your upper back. These are the muscles you use to pull your arms in toward you.

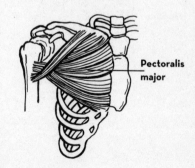

Pectoralis major

Your trapezius muscles (see Figure 7.3) are large, triangle-shaped muscles that run from just below your skull on either side of your neck, along the top of your scapula and down to your spine. They help support your head as well as your shoulders. The upper trapezius muscles assist in the elevation of the arm, the midtrapezius muscles pull shoulders toward the spine, and the lower trapezius muscles help keep your scapula close to your spine.

Deep Muscles

The deep muscles are equally important to good shoulder function. Because they are so close to the bones, the deep muscles help to stabilize the joints, keeping them in proper alignment when the larger muscles are executing movement. When you move your arm in any direction, your deep muscles are working just as hard as your larger muscles.

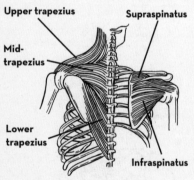

Figure 7.3

Upper trapezius

Supraspinatus

Mid-trapezius

Lower trapezius

Infraspinatus

But probably because you can't see them and because many people have never studied anatomy, very few of my clients understand how crucial it is to strengthen the deep muscles of their shoulders, so they rarely exercise them during their workouts.

In fact, I often find that when someone has strained a larger muscle, it is because their deeper, stabilizing muscles are weak and haven't been able to do their job of supporting the shoulder joints during movement.

If the deep muscles of the shoulder are exercised regularly along with the larger muscles, you will vastly improve how you move your upper body and significantly decrease your risk of injury.

Three of the more important deep muscle groups in your shoulder are the rotary cuff, the serratus anterior and the rhomboids. The rotary cuff muscles surround the shoulder joint and humerus, and help to support your joints. Three rotary cuff muscles that are often very tight, leading to many common injuries, are the supraspinatus (see Figure 7.3), the infraspinatus (see Figure 7.3), and the subscapularis (see Figure 7.4).

The serratus anterior muscles hold the scapula against your rib cage, both front and back. They work with your lower trapezius muscles to keep your scapula in its proper position close to the spine. When the serratus anterior muscles are weak, the lower part of the shoulder no longer stays anchored to the rib cage and begins to protrude, like wings. This very common condition, known as wing scapula, can be alleviated by strengthening the serratus anterior and lower trapezius muscles.

Figure 7.4

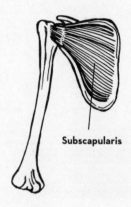

Subscapularis

The rhomboids are attached to the inner borders of the scapula. They pull the shoulders toward the spine and, when strong, work to improve your posture and, importantly, keep you from getting rounded shoulders.

At the end of this chapter are a number of excellent exercises that will help you strengthen these deep muscles. You will be amazed to see how much better you look and feel when these muscles are as strong and flexible as your lats and pecs.

Ligaments, Tendons, and Bursae

The muscles and bones that make up your shoulder joints would be helpless without the little soldiers that support them. The ligaments, which attach the bones to one another, the tendons, which attach the muscles to the bones, the cartilage, which enhances the depth of the joints, and the bursae, which cushion the joints, are all essential to efficient shoulder movement.

When your shoulder muscles are equally strong and flexible, all these components of your shoulder perform efficiently and painlessly.

But when you have weak or tight muscles, usually the result of overuse of some muscles and atrophy of others, the ligaments, tendons, bursae, and cartilage that assist in body mechanics often become strained. This is when injuries occur and pain results.

PAINS IN THE NECK

When you have bad posture, it's not just the muscles of your shoulder girdle that suffer, but your neck muscles as well. A number of neck muscles attach at the top of the shoulder, and poor posture can shorten these muscles, creating tension in the neck.

Limited mobility, muscle tightness, and pain are some of the more common neck maladies that can be remedied by stretching and strengthening the muscles of the neck.

Check Your Neck

Normal range of motion for the neck includes being able to rotate your head from side to side so that you can see behind you, extend, or tilt, your head back, and flex, or tilt, your head down so that your chin touches your chest. If you can't move your neck in these directions easily and without pain, you could have tight and weak neck muscles. Learning a few facts about your neck anatomy will help you understand how you can improve your neck mobility through stretching and strengthening exercises.

Neck Bones and Muscles

The neck includes seven bones that are part of the cervical spine and many muscles—deep muscles that sit very close to the bones of the neck and superficial muscles that lie farther away from the skeleton. All these muscles work together to support your head and enable mobility in the head and neck.

Among the deeper muscles are the scalene, longus, and levator muscles. These muscle groups allow you to lift your shoulders, rotate your neck, tilt your head from side to side, and drop your head forward over your chest. Of these muscles, the levators (see Figure 7.5) are notorious as pain sites. The levator muscles allow you to elevate your shoulders, but so many people keep their shoulders elevated because of daily work habits or tension that these muscles are often very tight, pulling the shoulder up and out of alignment. This causes the tendons surrounding the top of the humerus to become compressed and leads to pain.

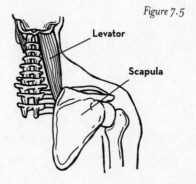

Figure 7.5

Levator

Scapula

People rarely think about exercising the deep muscles of the neck because they don't understand how important it is to keep them strong and flexible. As a result, these deep muscles are often weak and tight, which not only contributes to poor posture and tension in the neck but creates unhealthy strains on your shoulder joints.

The superficial muscles in the neck work with the deeper muscles to create movement. There are a number of these muscles, including the trapezius muscles (see Figure 7.3), but one set of muscles that causes trouble to many people are the sternocleidomastoids (see Figure 7.6). These muscles enable you to rotate your head and tilt it from side to side. If you have trouble turning your head around to look behind you, it's likely that these muscles are very tight, and you need to begin a stretching program to return them to their normal resting length.

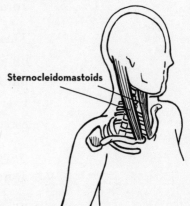

Figure 7.6

Sternocleidomastoids

If you are suffering from neck pain, it is often these and other muscles in the neck that are tight and/or weak. The exercises at the end of the chapter will go a long way toward improving your neck mobility and easing tension.

WHEN SHOULDERS GO SOUR

While accidents and congenital abnormalities can be the cause of shoulder injuries, many common shoulder injuries are created by imbalances in the strength of the muscles of the shoulder, which result in strains on all the components that make up the mechanism. Serious problems can include tears in the shoulder muscles, erosion of the cartilage that protects the joints, and dislocations in the shoulder joints, all of which can require surgery.

More common among my clients, however, are ailments that can often be significantly relieved by targeted exercise programming.

Tendinitis, Bursitis, and Impingement Syndrome

These painful conditions can occur separately or in combination when any of the shoulder muscles are weak or tight, putting strain on the other components of the shoulder. Exercises that stretch tight muscles and strengthen weak muscles can do a lot to relieve these conditions.

Tendinitis

When the tendons that connect the muscles to the shoulder bones are squeezed or pulled out of place by imbalances of strength and flexibility of the muscles, they can become inflamed, causing terrible pain when you move your arm. This is *tendinitis*. Also causing tendinitis is the aging process. Tendons can become less flexible as we get older, making them more prone to injury.

Tendinitis is common in the tendons that lie at the top of your shoulder, between the top of the humerus and the acromioclavicular joint, in the tendons of the rotary cuff muscles that surround the shoulder joint, and in the tendons of the biceps, just below your shoulder at the top of your arm.

Bursitis

There are a number of bursae in the shoulder, small, fluid-filled sacs that act as cushions, reducing friction between the tendons and bones and absorbing the shocks placed on the joints during movement. When, like tendons, these become compressed by imbalances of strength in the muscles of the shoulder, they can no longer function properly, making it painful to execute movement. This is called *bursitis*.

Shoulder Impingement

Tendons from the rotary cuff muscles can become thickened by inflammation and can get wedged under the acromioclavicular joint. When this happens, lifting your arm can become very painful, if not impossible, and you have *shoulder impingement*.

Arthritis

Degenerative wear and tear of the muscles, tendons, and ligaments of the shoulder can cause inflammation throughout the shoulder joint. This condition often compromises the range of motion in your shoulders and arms, and can be the cause of considerable pain.

Frozen Shoulder

When someone suffers an injury to the shoulder, such as getting hit in sports or falling, there can be swelling and inflammation at the site, which can cause adhesions of tissue to grow in between the joint. This inhibits the flow of synovial fluid that acts as a lubricant between the bone and socket. When this happens, the shoulder can become very stiff and painful, and movement can be limited to the point where someone can't lift his arm. This is called *frozen shoulder*.

SHAPING UP YOUR SHOULDERS AND NECK

Following are a series of strengthening and stretching exercises to get your shoulders back into shape and reduce tension in your neck. If office work has given you rounded shoulders, tight chest muscles, and a forward-tilting head, doing all these exercises daily will dramatically improve your posture and reduce any pain you may have.

Strengthening Exercises for the Shoulder

Strengthening and stretching all the muscles of your neck and shoulder will help you maintain good posture no matter what you do all day.

Shoulder Squeezes

This exercise strengthens your rhomboids and trapezius muscles, which help to maintain good posture.

1. Lie facedown on the floor, forehead on a folded towel, arms at your sides. (See Figure 7.7.)

2. Push your shoulders down and away from your ears, squeeze them together up toward your spine. (See Figure 7.8.)

3. Do two sets of 20 repetitions, adding a third set when it gets easier.

IMPORTANT: Think of melting your shoulders down into the back pockets of your pants.

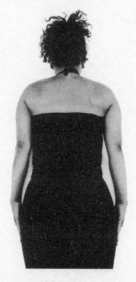

Figure 7.7

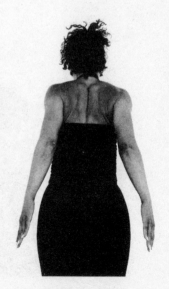

Figure 7.8

Shoulder Squeezes Progression

This exercise helps to remedy round shoulders.

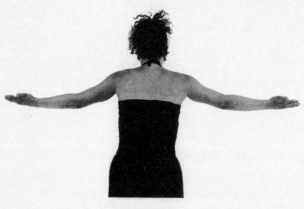

Figure 7.9

1. Lie facedown on the floor, forehead on a folded towel, arms straight out from the sides of your body, like airplane wings, thumbs pointing up to the ceiling. (See Figure 7.9.)

2. Anchor your shoulders down away from your ears and squeeze them together as you lift your arms. (See Figure 7.10.)

3. Do two sets of 20 repetitions, adding a third set when it gets easier.

IMPORTANT: Concentrate on keeping your shoulders down as you lift your arms.

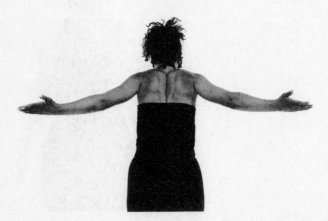

Figure 7.10

Shoulder Squeeze with Physio Ball

This exercise strengthens the rhomboids and lats.

1. Kneel in front of the physio ball with your legs apart. Extend your arms, resting your hands on the ball. (See Figure 7.11.)

2. Push down on the ball as you pull your elbows toward your waist. (See Figure 7.12.)

3. Squeeze shoulders together. Release

4. Do three repetitions of 10.

IMPORTANT: Press down on the ball throughout the exercise.

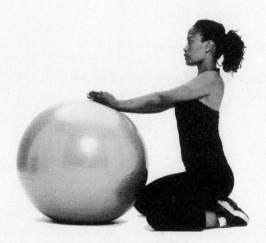

Figure 7.11

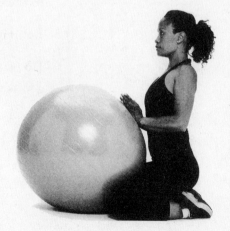

Figure 7.12

Angel

If you have pain in the lower part of your shoulder, your lower trapezius may be weak as a result of poor posture. This exercise strengthens the lower trapezius as well as the rhomboids and the rear deltoids.

1. Sit on a chair or physio ball. Bring your arms together, elbows, forearms, and hands touching as if in prayer. Your elbows should be bent at a right angle and held just below your collarbone. (See Figure 7.13.)

2. Open your arms out to your sides, keeping elbows bent—picture yourself as the strong man at the circus who stands with his arms up flexing his muscles. (See Figure 7.14.)

3. Squeeze your shoulders together, anchoring them down away from your ears, as if you were crushing a can between your shoulder blades.

4. Lower your elbows to the waist while lifting your chest up to the ceiling. (See Figure 7.15.)

5. Return to starting position. (See Figure 7.16.)

6. Do two sets of 20 repetitions, adding a third set when it gets easier.

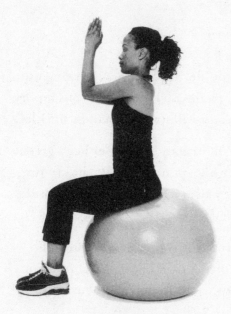

Figure 7.13

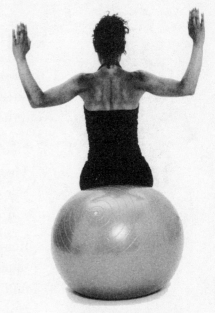

Figure 7.14

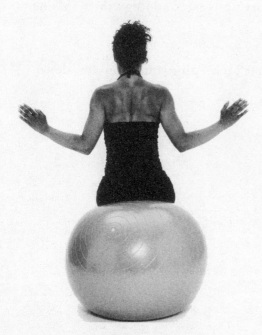

Figure 7.15

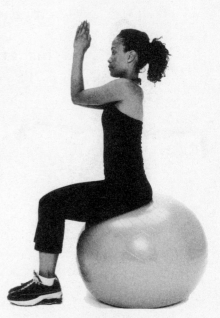

Figure 7.16

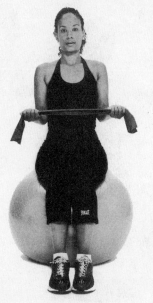

Figure 7.17

External Rotation

To protect yourself from shoulder injury when working out, you need strong rotary cuff muscles that will be able to support your shoulder joint. This exercise will strengthen these muscles.

1. Sit on a chair or physio ball, or stand. Using either a green Thera-Band latex band or one-pound weights, hold your elbows at the sides of your waist with palms facing up, as if you're holding a tray. (See Figure 7.17.)

2. Rotate your hands away from the center of your body, squeezing your shoulder blades together. Concentrate on pulling your shoulders down and anchoring them away from your ears. (See Figure 7.18.)

3. Do two sets of 20 repetitions each, adding a third set when it gets easier.

IMPORTANT: Concentrate on keeping your shoulders down.

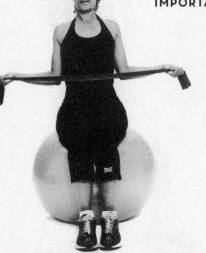

Figure 7.18

Serratus Push

If your shoulder is winging out of your back, you need to strengthen your serratus anterior muscles, which anchor your scapula to the rib cage. This strengthening exercise will help.

1. Stand facing a wall. Put your hands, palms flat, against the wall at shoulder level. Your arms should be straight, elbows locked.

2. Round your shoulders, pushing into the wall with your hands. Imagine making a camel hump with your upper back. (See Figure 7.19.)

3. Squeeze your shoulders together toward the spine, keeping elbows straight. (See Figure 7.20.)

4. Do two sets of 20 repetitions each, adding a third when it gets easier.

IMPORTANT: Don't let your shoulders inch up around your neck while doing this exercise, and remember to keep your elbows locked.

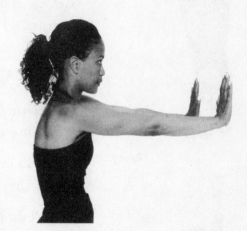

Figure 7.19

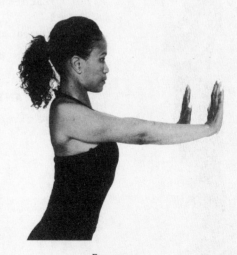

Figure 7.20

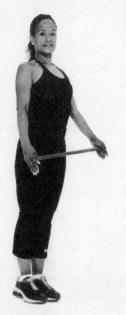

Flexibility Exercises for the Shoulder

People often lose flexibility in their neck and shoulders without even knowing it. Only gradually do they discover they can't swing their arms freely, reach for something without pain, or turn their head the way they used to. These exercises will ensure you will be able to turn your head to see your kids in the backseat of the car. They are just as important as strengthening exercises for total body fitness.

Cane Exercise

This exercise will help you if you have limited range of motion and stiffness in the shoulder joint.

Figure 7.21

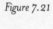

1. Hold a broom or other long stick with one hand and cup the other hand over the end of the pole. (See Figure 7.21.)

2. With the hand holding the pole held straight down at 6 o'clock, slowly push the pole so that the other hand reaches from 9 o'clock to 12 o'clock. (See Figure 7.22.)

3. Repeat eight times on each side, or as many times as needed until you feel the muscle releasing.

IMPORTANT: Go only as far as is comfortable, increasing your range of motion slowly and without pain.

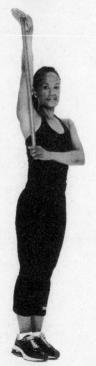

Figure 7.22

Chest Stretch with Rope or Towel

This exercise stretches chest muscles that have been tightened by poor posture. You can do the exercise either standing or sitting.

1. Sit on a chair or physio ball, with legs hip width apart, good posture, shoulders down.

2. With your arms straight up overhead and a little more than shoulder width apart, hold a rope or towel between your hands. (See Figure 7.23.)

3. Keeping your arms straight, reach behind you, feeling a comfortable stretch in your chest. (If you can't lift your arms over your head, increase the distance between your arms as you hold the rope or towel.) (See Figure 7.24.)

4. Hold for three to four seconds and repeat five times.

IMPORTANT: Keep shoulders down. Maintain a comfortable tension on the stretch and ease into a deeper stretch as you can.

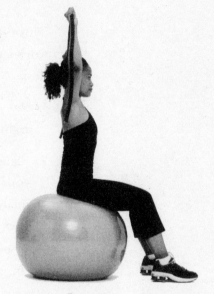

Figure 7.23

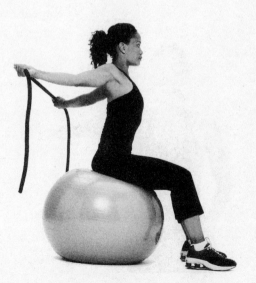

Figure 7.24

Shoulder Capsule Stretch

This exercise releases tense shoulder muscles, a very common workday hazard. You can do this exercise while sitting at your desk.

1. Put your left arm out to the side, holding your elbow at a right angle at the level of your collarbone. (See Figure 7.25.)

2. Place your right hand on your left elbow and slowly move your arm across your chest, using your right hand to gently push the arm as far as possible to the opposite shoulder. (See Figure 7.26.) You should feel this on the outside of your shoulder as the movement releases any tightness in the shoulder joint.

3. Repeat eight to ten times, or as many times as needed until you feel the muscle releasing.

4. Repeat exercise with your right arm.

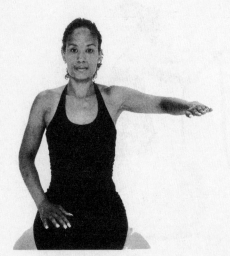

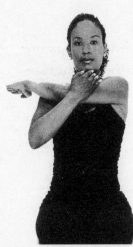

IMPORTANT: Concentrate on holding your shoulder down.

Figure 7.25

Figure 7.26

Sharman Stretch

This exercise opens the chest and helps maintain good posture.

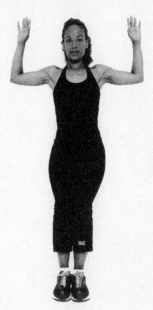

1. Stand with your back against a wall, with knees slightly bent. Keeping shoulders down, put your elbows, forearms, and the back of your hands flat against the wall at shoulder level. (See Figure 7.27.)

2. Slowly slide your hands overhead, keeping your shoulders and arms along the wall. (See Figure 7.28.)

3. Slide your arms back to the starting position.

4. Repeat eight to ten times, or as many times as you need to feel the muscles releasing.

Figure 7.27

IMPORTANT: Keep your shoulders down as you do this exercise.

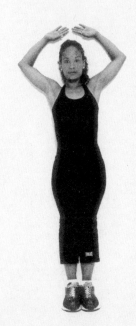

Figure 7.28

Shoulder Extension Stretch

This deeply satisfying stretch for the front muscles of the shoulder, called the anterior deltoids, opens up the chest.

1. Stand with your arms clasped behind your back. Keeping your arms straight, lift them, with your pinkies facing up, toward the ceiling as far as is comfortable.

2. Repeat eight to ten times or as many times as needed until you feel the muscle releasing.

IMPORTANT: Stand with good posture, looking straight ahead. Do not look down.

Flexibility Exercises for the Neck

Neck muscles are almost always too tight, so everyone can benefit from these exercises. You can do these exercises every day, at work or at home, to relax your neck to compensate for the strains of your daily activities.

Upper Trapezius

If you carry heavy shoulder bags, chances are your neck and shoulder muscles are tense. This exercise will release the tension in the neck.

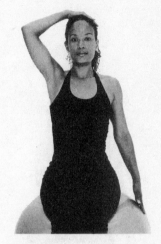

Figure 7.29

1. Sit or stand, keeping your shoulders down and your chest open and maintaining good posture. Put your right hand overhead, placing your palm on the top left side of your head. (See Figure 7.29.)

2. Using your hand, gently tilt your head to the right side, feeling the stretch in the neck muscles on your left side. (See Figure 7.30.)

3. Repeat up to eight times.

4. Repeat exercise on the other side to stretch the neck muscles on your right side.

IMPORTANT: Maintain good posture to get full benefit from this exercise.

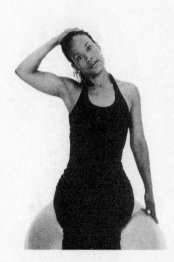

Figure 7.30

Levator Muscle Stretch

This stretches the levator muscles in the back of the neck and is a great exercise for someone who's on the phone all day.

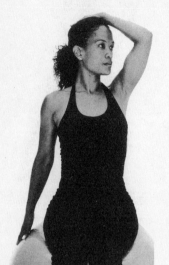

1. Sit upright, shoulders down, maintaining good posture, left arm on top of head, as in photo. (See Figure 7.31.)

2. Using your hand, as in the photo, rotate your head toward your left shoulder, aiming your chin toward your armpit and feeling the stretch in the muscles of your neck. (See Figure 7.32.)

3. Repeat up to eight times.

4. Return your head to the upright position and repeat the exercise on the other side, rotating your head toward your right shoulder.

Figure 7.31

5. Repeat up to eight times.

IMPORTANT: Keep your shoulders down.

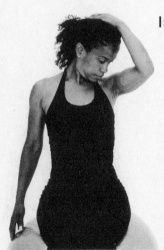

Figure 7.32

Neck Extensor Stretch

This stretches the often tight muscles in the back of the neck.

1. Sit upright, shoulders down, maintaining good posture, with your hands clasped behind your head. (See Figure 7.33.)

2. Without moving your shoulders, use your hands to gently pull your head downward toward your chest. (See Figure 7.34.)

3. Repeat up to eight times.

IMPORTANT: Make sure you keep your shoulders down when you clasp your hands behind your head.

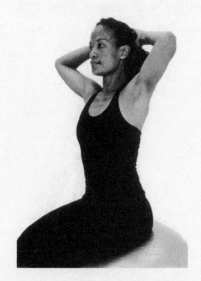

Figure 7.33

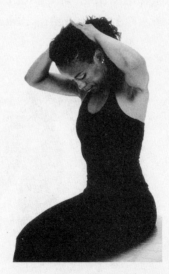

Figure 7.34

Head Nods

This is another easy stretching exercise for the neck muscles that you can do anywhere.

1. Sit, clasping your hands behind your back, keeping your shoulders down and your head turned to the side. (See Figure 7.35.)

2. Drop your head into your chest and nod up and down, moving your head to your right side as you nod. (See Figure 7.36.)

3. Nodding, return your head to the center, and repeat nods to the left side. (See Figure 7.37.)

4. Repeat up to eight times.

IMPORTANT: Keep your mouth closed. People often unconsciously open and shut their mouth when doing this exercise instead of stretching their neck muscles.

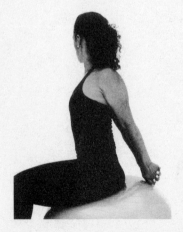
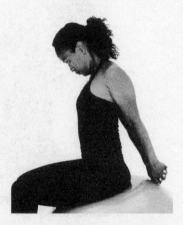
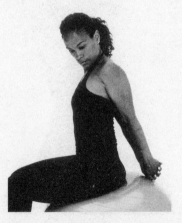

Figure 7.35   *Figure 7.36*   *Figure 7.37*

8

Elbows, Wrists, and Ankles—It's the Little Things That Count

It's amazing and depressing how much the smaller parts of the body can bother us. Occasional twinges in the wrists and elbows can gradually become dull aches or flashpoints of pain when we do the simplest, everyday tasks, such as moving a computer mouse on its pad or turning a doorknob. Ankles, too, can be a source of minor annoying twinges or pain so that you find yourself compromising your activities to avoid discomfort.

While many injuries to these extremities are caused by things that just happen—falls during sports, household accidents and the like—the way we use our bodies every day contributes mightily to problems with ankles, wrists, and elbows.

THE WRONGS WE DO
TO WRISTS AND ELBOWS

When I have clients with elbow and wrist pain who haven't just had a fall from Rollerblading or slammed their car door on their hand, the first two things I do are to check their posture and ask what they do during the day.

Poor Posture

It's no surprise that poor posture affects your shoulder muscles, but many people don't know that shoulder misalignment can lead to problems with your arms, especially your elbow joints. A number of arm muscles, like your biceps (see Figure 8.1) and triceps (see Figure 8.2), originate from the shoulder or cross the shoulder joint. They then run the length of your upper arm and are inserted at the elbow. When you have rounded shoulders, these muscles are affected, which can compromise the mechanics of the elbow joint.

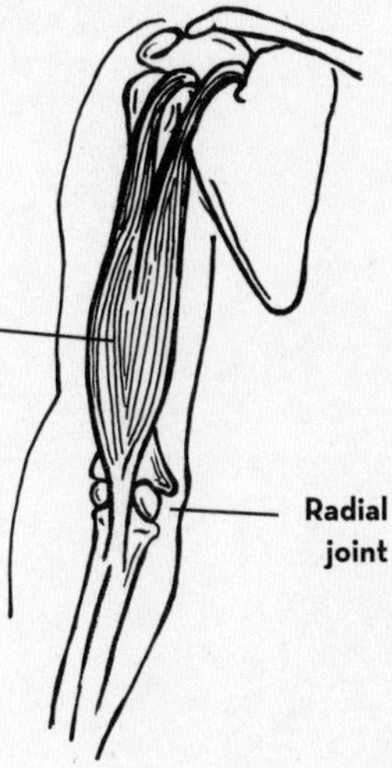

When this happens, it's not just the muscles of your arm that are affected, but the ligaments and tendons that surround them as well. Tight or overstretched muscles compress and strain the elbow joint, creating inflammation and pain in the ligaments and tendons that surround the joint.

Many things can cause elbow problems, but you should always be aware of the significant trickle-down effect of poor posture on the function of your elbow joint.

The trickle-down problems of the shoulder don't extend to the wrist, however. Most wrist problems can be traced to weaknesses in the muscles of the hands. It is these muscles that control the ability to flex and extend the fingers and stabilize the wrist joint.

Repetitive Movements

Using the same muscles every day without strengthening them for their function is another big reason for arm and wrist problems. Very often a client will complain about pain in her wrist or elbow or thumb and doesn't realize that she's simply suffering from muscle fatigue. It might seem like using a muscle over and over again would strengthen it, but that's not true. A muscle becomes strengthened when you train it to increase

Figure 8.1

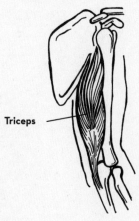

Biceps

Radial joint

Figure 8.2

Triceps

the amount of weight and use it can bear. In fact, the more you use a muscle in your daily activities, the more you need to strengthen it to keep up with the work it does. If you don't, the muscles get tired, and when they get tired, they get tight, which can cause pain.

A major league baseball pitcher would never go out on the mound without properly training his shoulder muscles to keep them strong and flexible for the extraordinary work he's asking of them.

It's the same with any of the muscles in the body. Your work might not put you on national television like major league pitcher Randy Johnson, but just because you spend your day chopping vegetables for hours at a time as a line cook or tapping away at a keyboard doesn't mean you're using your muscles any less than Randy. You're probably using them more, in fact, since you don't get the winters off.

WHAT'S INSIDE YOUR ARM

The bones, ligaments, and tendons that make up the arms work together with amazing synchrony to allow a wide range of movement, especially when all the muscles are strong and flexible.

Bones and Joints

The three primary bones of the arm are the humerus, which is the upper arm bone, running from the shoulder to the elbow, and the radius and ulna, two bones of the lower arm, which attach at the elbow and wrist. The radius is located on the inner part of your arm, in line with your thumb, and the ulna runs along the outer part of the forearm, in line with the pinkie.

In your lower arm, the radius and ulna meet at the bones of the hand, called carpals, at the wrist joint. (See Figure 8.3.) Here, too, there are two components to the joint to allow flexible movement between the hand and the two bones of the forearm. The radiocarpal joint is the site where the radius meets the bones of the hand, and the midcarpal joint allows you to flex your hand up and down.

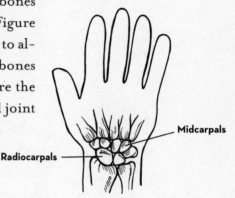

Radiocarpals

Midcarpals

Figure 8.3

Muscles

Almost everyone knows where their biceps are—in the front of the upper arm—and can locate their triceps, which run down the back of the upper arm from shoulder to elbow. These are the muscles that give you the power to flex and extend your elbows, and most people exercise them because they yearn for toned upper arms.

But there are other muscles that help to navigate the elbow, wrist, and hand. The supinator muscle runs along the outer part of your elbow to your hand and is used whenever you turn your palm up. The pronator muscles are located on the inside of your arm and are needed to turn your palm down, which is called pronation.

You use your pronator and supinator muscles continually throughout the day with any rotation, from opening a door or unscrewing a jar top to tightening a pipe fitting with a wrench. Strengthening these muscles for the work you do will significantly reduce your risk for injury.

Ligaments and Tendons

There are a number of ligaments in the elbows and wrists whose job is to connect the bones in the arm and hand. Along with the muscles that surround the bones, the ligaments help provide stability to the elbow and wrist joints. But if the muscles in the arm are tight and weak and not conditioned, the ligaments can become strained, causing pain and sometimes injury during movement.

Like the elbow, the wrist has a number of ligaments and tendons that work together with the bones in the lower forearm and hand to assure efficient movement of the wrist and hand. When they become strained, however, often as a result of overuse injuries, the tendons and then the ligaments swell, causing pain and sometimes injury.

WRIST AND ELBOW MALADIES

A few of the more common wrist and elbow injuries are listed below to give you a basic idea of why you're feeling discomfort or pain.

Epicondylitis

At the lower end of your humerus are your epicondyles—smooth, cartilage-like tissue that helps ensure the fluid movement of the elbow joint. When they become irritated or inflamed, often because of overuse of the muscles in the arm, they can cause pain. The lateral epicondyle, located on the outer side of the elbow, often becomes strained when tennis players take to the court without strengthening their muscles for their sport, or if they have poor form. The medial epicondyle is on the inner elbow and is a common site for strains among deconditioned weekend golfers, because the golf stroke calls upon the muscles on the inside of the arm.

Inflammation of the Flexor Tendons/Tennis Elbow

There are approximately 15 muscles in the forearm that surround the elbow and wrist, and they are frequently subjected to heavy use, particularly in racquet sports. When they are not conditioned for these activities, the muscles are pushed beyond their level of strength, which is called overuse. When this occurs, the tendons that attach the muscles to the bones try to compensate for muscle weaknesses and become inflamed and swollen, causing sharp pain during movement. Tennis elbow is one familiar example of this malady, but many activities can cause inflammation of the tendons in the forearm.

Carpal Tunnel Syndrome

This very common overuse injury that plagues many people who use keyboards at work has thankfully received a lot of attention and is now often prevented by putting a pad below the keyboard so typists can keep their wrists straight when they type. But if you find that your hands are numb or if you have a tingling sensation in your hands and wrists, you could suffer from this syndrome. It is caused by inflammation of the tendons in the wrists, which press on the nerves that go into the wrists. The nerves, which travel into the wrist through a tunnel called the carpal tunnel, then become impinged, causing the symptoms described above. Exercises and proper ergonomics at the workplace can alleviate this problem.

THE LOWDOWN ON THE ANKLE

Many ankle problems I see among my clients are due to weak or tight muscles and poor balance. Wearing shoes without proper support, having to stand for long periods of time, and being overweight can all contribute to muscle weakness in the ankle.

This isn't to say all ankle pain and injuries are your fault, as accidents can happen to anyone—just ask any of the huge number of people who show up in doctors' offices with ankle sprains. But since many injuries happen when a person loses his footing, either in sports or by stepping on an uneven surface, the stronger your muscles are and the better balance you have, the better your chances of regaining your footing without falling.

Learning more about how the ankle works and understanding how to exercise can go a long way toward stabilizing your ankle joint.

Ankle Bones and Joints

Your ankle is the meeting place of your two lower leg bones, the tibia and fibula, and two of the bones of your foot. The talus is on the top of your foot, and the calcaneus is in your heel. These bones make up your ankle joint, a hinge joint, which gives you the ability to flex and extend and rotate your foot.

Ankle Muscles, Ligaments, and Tendons

Your ankle joints are supported by a number of muscles that surround them and enable joint movement. Among them are the tibialis anterior, which runs along your shin and allows you to flex your toes off the floor, and the peroneal muscles, located on the outer side of your lower leg and giving you the ability to turn your foot in and out.

In the back of your lower leg are the calf muscles: the gastrocnemius muscles, which connect to the Achilles tendon, and the deeper soleus muscle. (See Figure 8.4.)

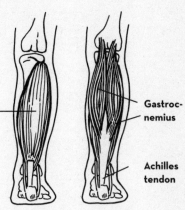

Figure 8.4

When these muscles are working properly, the ligaments and tendons that support the joint are also strong and flexible, and you have a very efficient package that allows you to walk easily.

Often, however, people will exercise to strengthen some of their lower leg muscles, particularly their calf muscles, but don't exercise those on the sides and front of their lower legs. In addition, they don't stretch their calf muscles properly, so that these muscles are often very tight. Having these weak and tight muscles can create balance problems and increase the risk of falling.

This is one reason why everyone's heard of the Achilles tendon, which is the largest tendon in the foot, connecting the heel to the muscle. When your muscles are strong and flexible and do their job of supporting your ankle and foot, your ligaments and tendons are anonymous, quietly supporting and stabilizing the muscles and bones.

But tight calf muscles combined with quick movements and poor form can put far too much strain on the Achilles tendon, pulling and overstretching the tendon and sometimes causing it to tear.

Strengthening and stretching all the muscles of your ankle will significantly improve your balance and allow all the parts of your legs, ankles, and feet to work efficiently so that you avoid pain and injury.

COMMON ANKLE PROBLEMS

The most common reason my clients hurt their ankles is that they're not strengthening all the muscles that surround the ankle joint. They have muscle weaknesses, which lead to balance problems. A series of balance exercises is very effective in strengthening the ankle joint and preventing falls. Below are simple explanations of some common ankle problems.

Ankle Sprains

An *ankle sprain* occurs when the ligaments connecting the bones of the ankle joint become strained or torn. This condition often occurs when the muscles surrounding the ankle are tight or weak, forcing the ligaments to take on more stress than they can handle. Exercises that increase the flexibility, strength, and endurance of the muscles in this area can go a long way toward preventing sprains.

Plantar Fasciitis

When you have shooting pains in your heel when you step out of bed in the morning, the doctor will often diagnose *plantar fasciitis,* which means the fascia, a sheath of fibrous tissue that runs from the heel to the ball of the foot, has become tight. During the day, you might not notice any problem because you are stretching the tissue when you walk, but when you are sedentary in bed at night, the fascia tightens up. This condition can be the result of improperly fitting shoes, being overweight, or repetitive stress from running. Rolling a rubber ball under your bare foot helps relieve this condition.

Shin Splints

This is another "tight" muscle problem affecting the muscles of the tibia, which are in the front of the lower leg. When these muscles are tight and you put a lot of weight on them, which happens, for instance, when runners run downhill, the muscles can't absorb the stress the way they would if they were flexible, so you feel pain. A good stretching program goes a long way toward preventing shin splints.

ELBOW, WRIST, AND ANKLE EXERCISES

Following are a number of excellent exercises for the elbows, wrists, and ankles. They include strengthening exercises to help you condition your body for any sports you like, as well as common workday tasks, and stretching exercises, which are helpful for those with overuse injuries. You can add these exercises to those with which you are already familiar: biceps and wrist curls and triceps extensions.

Elbow Stretch

This exercise is helpful for those suffering from tennis elbow, tendinitis, or epicondylitis.

1. Sit or stand with good posture, shoulders back and down. Keeping your arm straight and elbow locked, bring your right arm diagonally across your body. Close your right hand in a loose fist, and clasp it with your left hand. (See Figure 8.5.)

2. Flex your wrist inward by pushing down on your right hand with your left hand, feeling the stretch along the outside of your lower right arm. (See Figure 8.6.)

3. Do two or three times.

4. Repeat with the left arm.

IMPORTANT: Keep your arms straight, elbows locked, and hand in a loose fist.

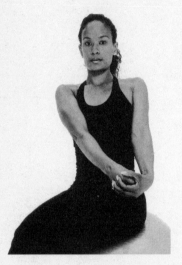

Figure 8.5

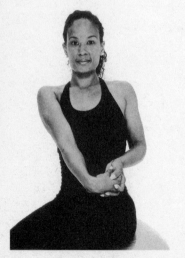

Figure 8.6

Stretch for the Muscles of the Forearm

This is a good exercise for people who work at a keyboard.

1. Sitting or standing, extend your right arm straight out in front of you, with your inner arm turned upward, at chest height. Make a loose fist. (See Figure 8.7.)

2. Flex your wrist toward you. Place your left hand over your fist and gently pull your right wrist into a stretch, using a comfortable tension. (See Figure 8.8.)

3. Repeat up to eight times.

4. Repeat exercise with the left arm.

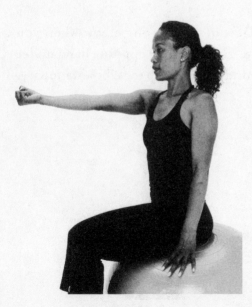

Figure 8.7

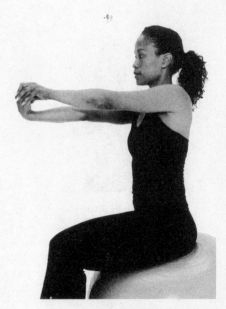

Figure 8.8

Supinator and Pronator

This elbow exercise strengthens the muscles you use to turn your palm up and down, useful in sports as well as in many daily tasks.

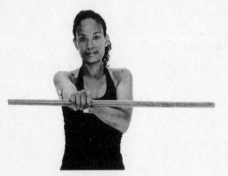

Figure 8.9

1. With your right arm straight out in front of you, hold a stick or light weight in your hand, palm facing down. (See Figure 8.9.)

2. Hold your right elbow with your left hand to keep your elbow stationary while you rotate your right forearm and wrist. (See Figure 8.10.)

3. Rotate your wrist so that your palm faces upward. (See Figure 8.11.)

4. Do three sets of 20 repetitions with each arm.

IMPORTANT: Do not rotate your elbow when you move your hand. Holding your opposite hand under your elbow reminds you to keep the elbow stationary.

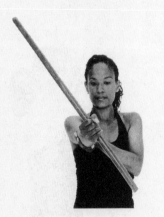

Figure 8.10

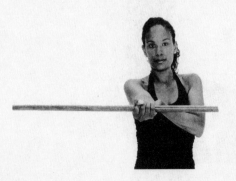

Figure 8.11

Ball Squeeze

This is an excellent exercise to stabilize and strengthen the muscles that run from the wrist to the elbow, helpful for those using a keyboard.

1. Sit with good posture, with your elbow bent at a right angle and tucked against your waist, your hand spread open in front of you holding a rubber handball. (See Figure 8.12.)

2. Squeeze the ball. (See Figure 8.13.)

3. Do three repetitions of 20 squeezes with each hand.

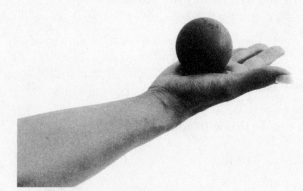

Figure 8.12

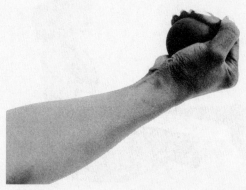

Figure 8.13

Ankle Strengthener

This exercise is a very good stretch for the gastrocnemius and soleus muscles.

1. Sit on the floor with good posture—back straight, shoulders down—right leg extended and left leg tucked under right leg.

2. Hook a Thera-Band elastic band around the ball of your right foot, creating tension against your foot. (See Figure 8.14.)

3. Point and flex your toes, pushing against the Thera-Band and feeling the stretch in your calf muscles. (See Figure 8.15.)

4. Do two or three sets of 20 repetitions.

5. Repeat with the left foot.

IMPORTANT: You can do this with your shoes on or off.

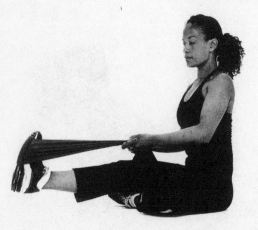

Figure 8.14

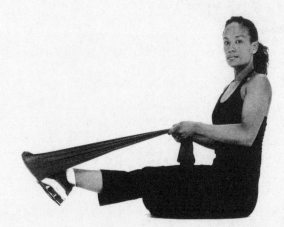

Figure 8.15

Heel Cord Stretch, Part 1

Many people don't know how to correctly stretch their calf muscles. This exercise does this and is excellent for runners both before and after running.

1. Sit on the floor, legs straight out in front of you, feet flexed, right foot on top of left foot, heel to toe. Put a towel or rope around your right foot. (See Figure 8.16.)

2. Keeping your back straight and maintaining good posture, lean forward over your leg. Flex your foot and, squeezing the muscles around your kneecap, pull your toes toward you with the towel. (See Figure 8.17.)

3. Hold for three seconds. Repeat eight to ten times until you feel a release.

4. Reverse position so that your left foot is on top of your right foot and repeat the exercise.

IMPORTANT: Keep back straight. Look for comfortable tension with this exercise, and ease up if you feel pain.

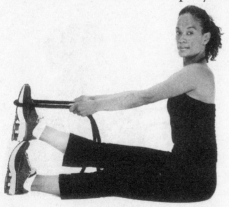

Figure 8.16

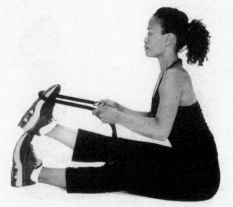

Figure 8.17

Heel Cord Stretch, Part 2

This exercise stretches your outer calf muscles.

1. Sit on the floor, legs straight out in front of you, feet flexed, right foot on top of left foot, heel to toe.

2. Put a towel on either side of your right foot. (See Figure 8.18.)

3. Rotate your right foot inward, as if you were pigeon-toed. Keeping your back straight and maintaining good posture, lean forward over the leg, and, keeping toes flexed and facing inward and squeezing the muscles around your kneecap, pull your toes toward you with the towel. (See Figure 8.19.)

4. Hold for three seconds. Repeat eight to ten times until you feel a release.

5. Repeat exercise with the left foot.

IMPORTANT: Look for comfortable tension with this exercise. Ease up if you feel pain.

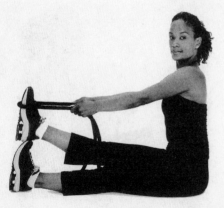

Figure 8.18

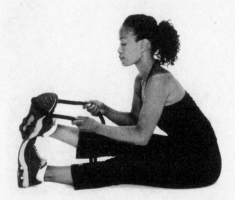

Figure 8.19

Ankle Alphabet

This is a good exercise for all the muscles that stabilize the ankle and helps you to balance.

1. Sit on the floor with your left knee bent and foot flat on the floor. Cross your right leg over your left leg. (See Figure 8.20.)

2. Using your right foot as a pointer, write the alphabet from A to Z with your toe. (See Figure 8.21.)

3. Repeat the alphabet twice with each foot.

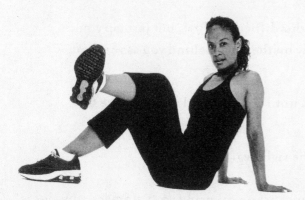

Figure 8.20

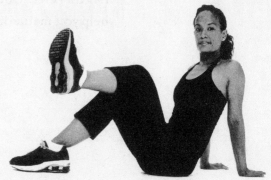

Figure 8.21

Ankle Balance

This strengthens the muscles that stabilize the ankle joint and significantly improves your balance.

1. Stand up straight, arms held out to your sides, feet underneath your body.

2. Bend your right knee slightly and lift your left foot off the floor, keeping your stomach muscles tight to help you maintain your balance.

3. When you feel stable, close your eyes and try to maintain your balance.

4. You will find this difficult at first, but just tap your left foot lightly on the floor behind you as you find your balance.

5. Time yourself until you can hold your balance for a minute.

6. Repeat with the right leg.

IMPORTANT: Concentrate on using your stomach muscles to help you maintain balance. It works.

9

Take Charge
of Your Body

Now that you have read about the different zones of your body and learned how your joints work and the importance of training them properly, it's time to step back and focus on your overall fitness program.

One of the unique strengths of my programming is teaching clients about joint health and how, through exercise, they can ensure better joint mechanics, move more efficiently, and prevent injury. But the reason my program has been so successful is that once my clients have a basic knowledge of their zones, I explain how crucial it is that these zones work together so the *whole* body is strong, flexible, and in proper alignment.

Strengthening the muscles around an aching knee is great, but if your posture is poor and your core muscles weak, you'll enjoy a temporary benefit to your knee but not the long-term improvement in your alignment that will keep you healthy and strong and reduce your risk for injury.

With that in mind, and knowing from my clients that creating an overall program from all the exercises I give them can be overwhelming, below is a sample workout that is beneficial to all the zones of the body and promotes good posture and alignment. If you combine these exercises with cardiovascular exercise and do them two or three times a week, you will feel and look dramatically better in a very short time. Your posture and balance will improve, you will look taller and thinner, and you will find that many of the annoying aches and pains that might be bothering you will disappear.

Each of these exercises is explained in earlier chapters, so I've put the photos here to guide you, as well as the page numbers if you need to refer back to written instruction. You can cut these pages out of the book and tape them on the wall to help you follow the routine. As you become more familiar with the workout, you can add other exercises from the book.

I have divided my usual hour workout into two half-hour sessions to give you some flexibility if you're short on time.

The workout includes excellent strengthening exercises for your core muscles, as well as basic strengthening and stretching exercises for all the postural groups. Note that there is a balance between strengthening and stretching exercises. Stretching is often neglected in the heat of exercise but is very important in helping the muscles stay healthy and flexible.

Your workout will exercise the muscles in your core, back, hips, knees, shoulders, and neck. These exercises emphasize the muscle groups that are most important to good posture and joint health, muscles groups that are often ignored in workouts, so you won't find more common exercises here. This doesn't mean that you should abandon your current exercise regimen, but that you should add these exercises to them to ensure overall strength and flexibility.

Each exercise has an explanation of what part of the body you're training and why so that you understand your workout and can tailor your exercises to your own activities.

The exercises should be executed with a comfortable tension and can be modified if they are too strenuous. I've explained how to do this in the written texts of the exercises. Nothing should hurt.

As you do the exercises, pay attention to which exercises are easier for you and which are more difficult. When an exercise is difficult, it's very often related to the fact that the muscles you're working are either weak or tight. This is a sign that you need to focus on strengthening or stretching these muscles.

Generally, my clients find that some muscles are stronger or weaker than others, that they have muscle tightness from not stretching properly, that one side of their bodies is stronger than the other, and that their balance isn't as good as they thought. You will probably make similar discoveries about yourself.

As you learn more about how your own body works, and combine that knowledge with the anatomy you've learned throughout this book, as well as the explanations provided with the exercises, you will gradually gain the confidence you need to take charge of your own body in a way you've probably never done before.

I've made this program very user-friendly. Because there are no machines and very few pieces of equipment, you can do it anywhere—at home in front of the television, in a hotel room, while the baby is napping. You have no excuse but to get ready to look and feel better fast!

Note: I've put the Neck Extensor Stretch, Standing Outer Hip Stretch, and Ankle Balance exercises in both workout routines because they address very common problems, but if you combine your sessions into one workout, you need to do these exercises only once.

Workout One

Trunk Flexion

This is a "standing crunch" that strengthens your stomach muscles. (See p. 38.)

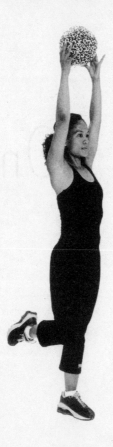

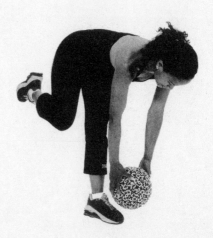

Hook Lying

This exercises the lower abdominal muscles and the muscles of the pelvic floor. (See p. 43.)

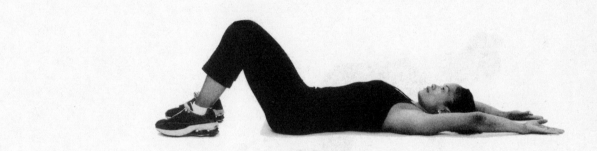

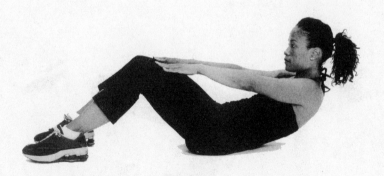

Quadruped

This is a therapeutic exercise for people with chronic back pain. It is designed to strengthen the muscles that stabilize the spine. (See p. 65.)

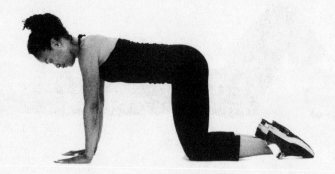

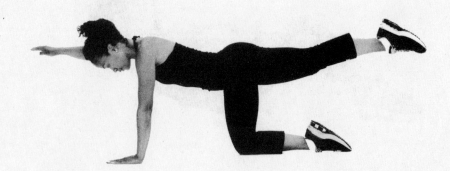

Step Ups

This is another way to strengthen the muscles that extend your knee. (See p. 109.)

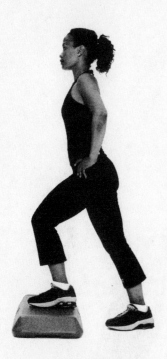

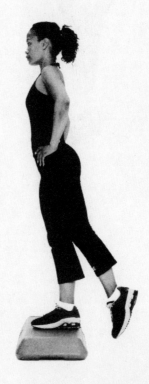

Standing Outer Hip Stretch

This exercise releases tension in the outer hip, which can sometimes contribute to a tight iliotibial band. (See p. 116.)

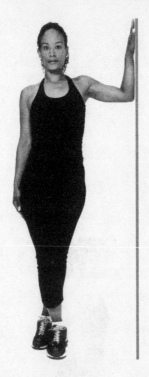

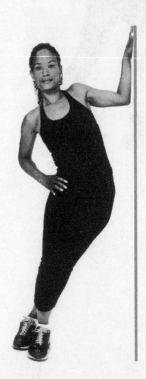

Seated Groin Stretch

This stretches the muscles in the front of your hips. (See p. 92.)

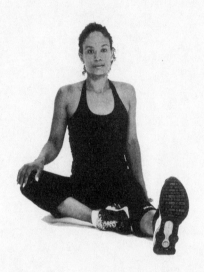

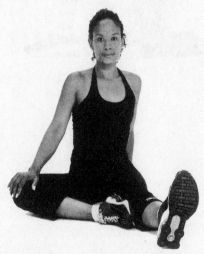

Hip Flexor/Psoas Stretch

This is an important exercise to stretch this often tight muscle and return it to its normal resting length. (See p. 62.)

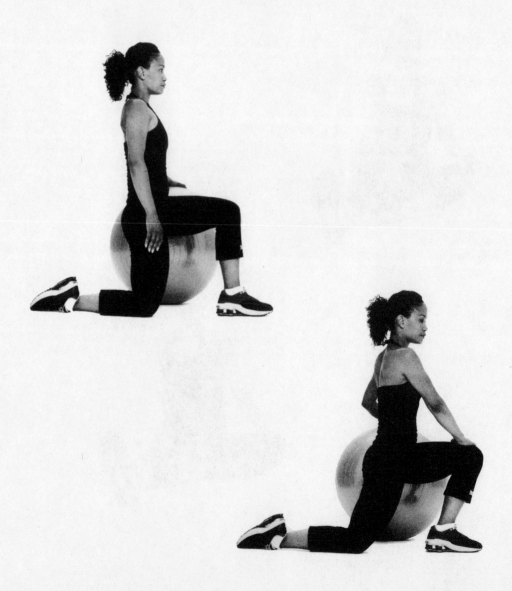

Trunk Flexion Stretch

This is a good stretch for the muscles of the lower spine. (See p. 60.)

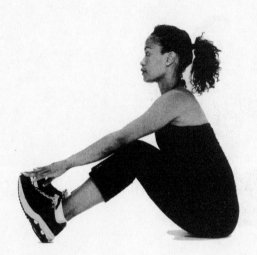

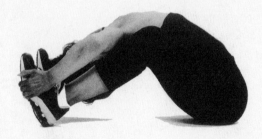

Heel Cord Stretch, Part 1

Many people don't know how to correctly stretch their calf muscles. This exercise does this and is excellent for runners both before and after running. (See p. 117.)

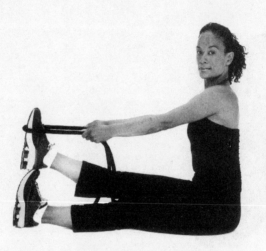

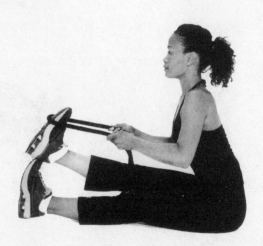

Shoulder Squeezes

This exercise strengthens your rhomboids and trapezius muscles, which help to maintain good posture. (See p. 135.)

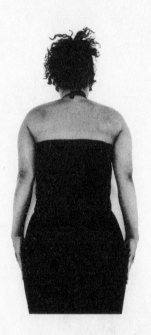

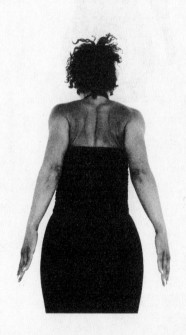

Levator Muscle Stretch

This stretches the levator muscles in the back of the neck and is a great exercise for someone who's on the phone all day. (See p. 148.)

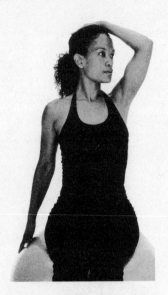

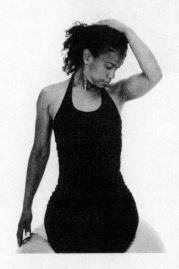

Neck Extensor Stretch

This stretches the often tight muscles in the back of the neck.
(See p. 149.)

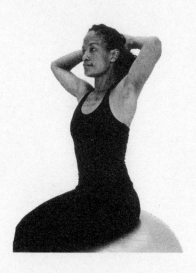

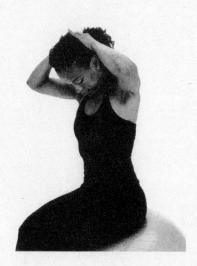

Ankle Balance

This strengthens the muscles that stabilize the ankle joint and
significantly improves your balance. (See p. 170.)

Workout Two

Lateral Flexion

This exercises the transverse abdominus.
(See p. 39.)

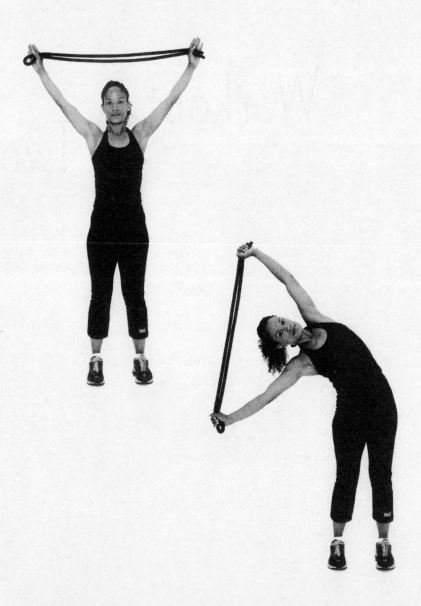

Lying Trunk Rotation

This exercise strengthens the obliques and rectus abdominus and other small muscles that stabilize the spine. (See p. 42.)

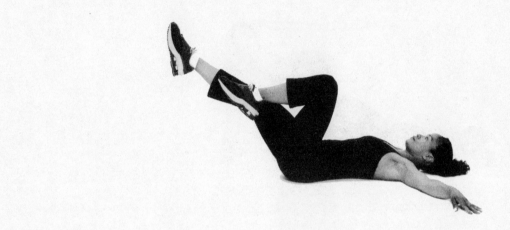

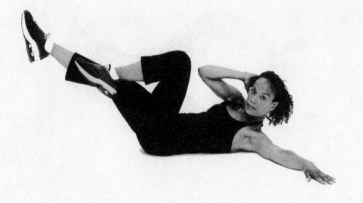

Clams

This exercise strengthens the outer muscles of the hip, as strong hip muscles help keep the knee in its proper position. (See p. 82.)

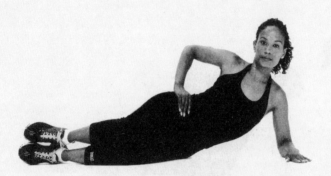

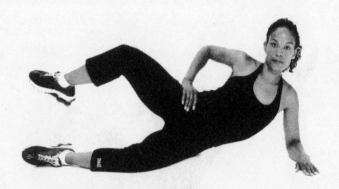

External Rotation with Abduction

This is an excellent exercise to strengthen the outer hip muscles, including the gluteus medius. (See p. 83.)

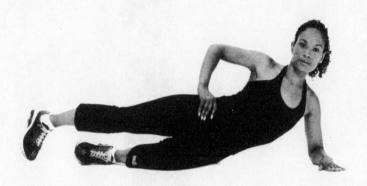

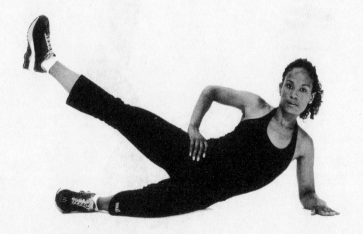

Step Downs

This will strengthen the leg muscles that help to bend, or flex, the knee. (See p. 110.)

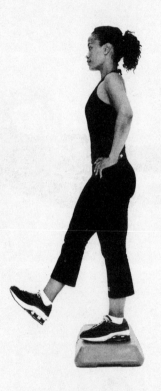

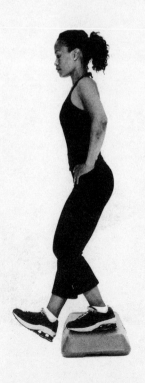

Standing Outer Hip Stretch

This exercise releases tension in the outer hip, which can sometimes contribute to a tight iliotibial band, described in chapter 6. (See p. 89.)

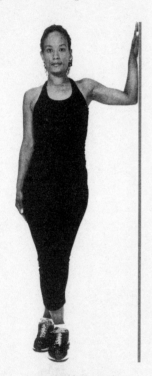

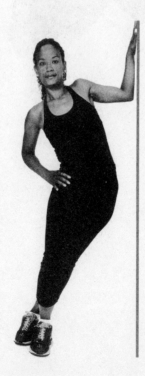

Trunk Flexion Stretch

This is a good stretch for the muscles of the lower spine.
(See p. 60.)

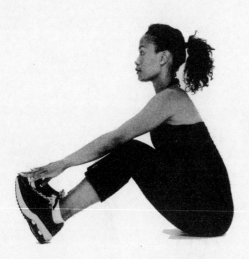

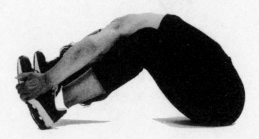

Quadratus Stretch

A good stretch for all the back muscles. (See p. 63.)

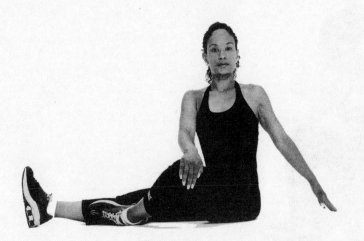

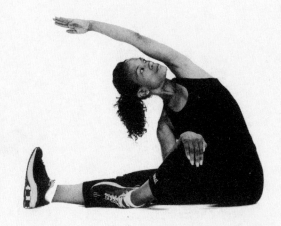

Quadriceps Stretch

This exercise helps reduce tension in the knees. (See p. 115.)

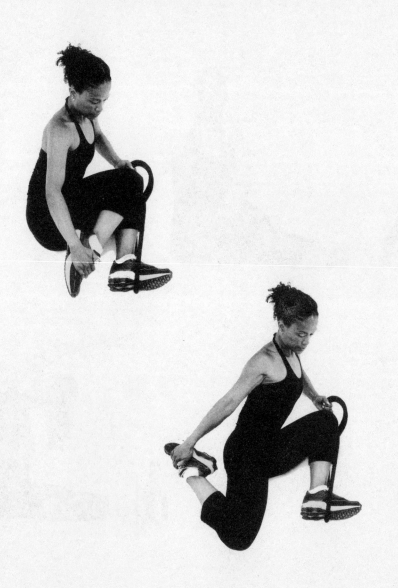

Shoulder Capsule Stretch

This exercise releases tense shoulder muscles, a very common workday hazard. You can do this exercise while sitting at your desk. (See p. 144.)

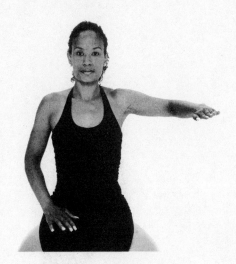

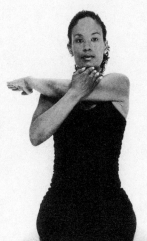

Neck Extensor Stretch

This stretches the often tight muscles in the back of the neck. (See p. 149.)

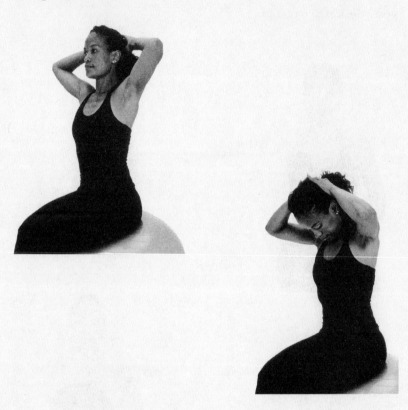

Ankle Balance

This strengthens the muscles that stabilize the ankle joint and significantly improves your balance. (See p. 170.)

10

Exercise
Intelligence

Now that you understand a little bit about how your body works, are aware of how you move, and know exercises that can keep you strong and flexible, you can be the architect of your own fitness.

You know that true fitness is far more than buff biceps and a flat stomach. It is a recognition of how beautifully the body is designed and how well it functions when we take care of it. It is understanding that it is up to you to learn enough about your own body mechanics so that you can exercise intelligently and enjoy a full range of movement throughout your lifetime.

WORKING OUT ON YOUR OWN

A good fitness program helps you maintain good posture, increases your flexibility and strength, and enables more efficient movement of your joints and muscles while reducing the risk of injury.

You can design a complete exercise program for yourself that includes:

- cardiovascular exercise to improve the strength of the heart and lungs and to control your weight;

- strengthening exercises for all your muscles, especially those that improve your posture and balance;

- targeted exercises that strengthen weak muscles and stretch tight muscles to ensure healthier joints and efficient movement;

- deep stretching at the end of a workout to return muscles to their normal resting length.

Most important, you know *why* all these areas are important to true fitness, and you have the skills to tailor a program to your own needs and to choose exercises that will keep you healthy and fit throughout your life.

WORKING WITH A TRAINER

If you work with a trainer or are thinking of doing so, what you've learned here will complement your workouts and help you communicate to the trainer your goals and specific needs.

Any trainer you work with should know at least as much as you do about the components of an intelligent exercise program. If she doesn't, you'll find out pretty fast.

Below are some guidelines to developing an efficient workout program. Knowing them will help you to communicate to a trainer your specific fitness needs and goals, and aid you in choosing a trainer who understands what you are trying to accomplish.

- Appreciate the importance of good posture, of strengthening the muscles of the core, of training for functionality.

- Understand that poor daily postural habits can compromise your movement. Identify them and exercise to correct those habits.

- Pay close attention to any pain or stiffness you feel either during a workout or outside the gym so that you can modify your exercise program if you need to. A trainer should know how to do this.

- Make sure you use the correct technique when exercising.

- Track your progress to ensure that you get the results you're looking for, both functionally and aesthetically.

FINALLY FIT

I hope you have a better understanding of your body and can use the knowledge you've gained to design a personalized workout that addresses all your fitness needs and keeps you healthy and pain-free for your lifetime.

Index

Numbers in italics indicate illustrations.